DATE DUE

OCLC/liooirPl	
H-2-10	
GAYLORD	PRINTED IN U.S.A.

THE ILLUSTRATED SURGERY GUIDE

20 common operations explained step-by-step

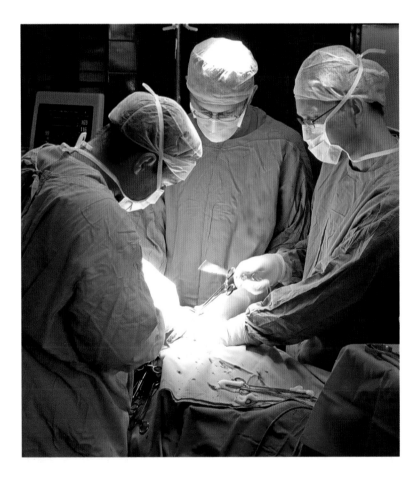

Quercus Publishing Plc
21 Bloomsbury Square
London
WC1A 2NS

First published in 2009

A catalog record of this book is available from the British Library

ISBN 978-1-84866-035-9

Printed and bound in China

10 9 8 7 6 5 4 3 2 1

NOTE TO READERS

The information contained in this book provides general guidance on preparing for surgery and what happens when a patient is taken into the operating theater. All hospitals, surgeons, and patients are different and you should obtain specific information relating to your own condition and operation from your healthcare provider.

This book is not a Do-It-Yourself guide to surgery. All operations are potentially life threatening and must be carried out by fully trained, medically qualified surgeons. None of the procedures described in this book should be attempted under any circumstances. The author and publisher cannot be held responsible for any adverse effects or consequences from the use or application of the information in this publication.

This book is not a substitute for professional medical or health care. The advice in this book is based on the training, expertise, and information available to the author. Where there is any question regarding the presence or treatment of any health condition, the author and publisher urge the readers to consult a qualified health professional.

Any research studies and institutions cited in this book should in no way be construed as an endorsement of anything in this book. The author and publisher expressly disclaim any responsibility for any adverse effects arising from the use or application of the information contained herein.

THE ILLUSTRATED SURGERY GUIDE

20 common operations explained step-by-step

Dr Sarah Brewer

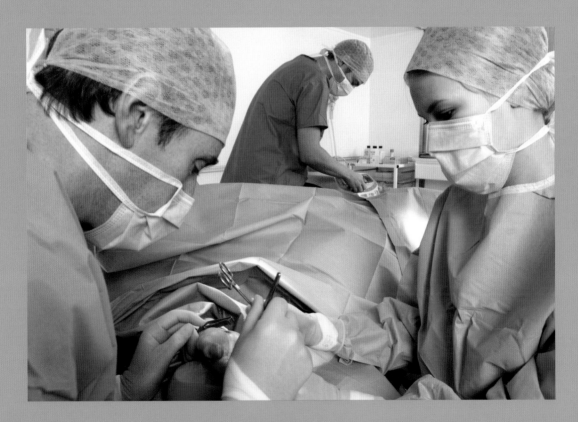

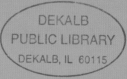
Quercus

CONTENTS

INTRODUCTION

The number of surgical procedures carried out in the United States every year is forecast to exceed 38 million in 2012 — around 10 million more than occurred in 2004. This trend is partly because of the development of new surgical techniques, and partly because more operations are now taking place in an inpatient setting — either in hospital-based "ambulatory" units or freestanding surgical centers.

The Illustrated Surgery Guide explains everything you need to know about the most common operations performed every year in the United States. The 20 procedures are featured in order with the most common first. Figures are based on data from the Agency for Healthcare Research and Quality National Statistics Database, and from the Ambulatory Surgery in the United States National Health Statistics Report published in 2009.

Each entry explains what the procedure is and why it may prove necessary. Green colored boxes provide additional surgical information, while blue boxes also contain general advice and supplementary information about the condition. An at-a-glance panel tells you if it can be performed as an outpatient, whether you need a general anesthetic, and what special tests are needed beforehand. This panel also tells you how long the surgery takes, how long you are likely to stay in hospital, and gives you an idea of the relative cost. Operations illustrated with one dollar sign 💲 are relatively cheap (typically less than $25,000) while those with five dollar signs 💲💲💲💲💲 are relatively expensive (typically above $100,000).

Unfortunately, all surgical operations entail some risk, especially those performed under general anesthetic. The general risks are discussed in the next section, while the specific risks associated with each operation are explained in the relevant chapter. The at-a-glance panel also tells you the expected mortality rate for the procedure.

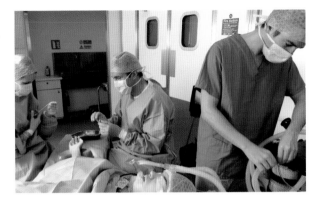

ABOVE A surgeon, anesthesiologist, and nurse prepare to perform an operation on the hand of a female patient.

How each operation is performed is fully explained in the Step-By-Step section, which is illustrated with pictures from real surgical procedures. This gives you an excellent idea of what to expect when having the operation — whether it involves an elective outpatient procedure or an emergency hospital admission. The chapters tell you about the risks and benefits of each operation, and about any alternative ways to manage your condition medically or surgically. Each section also outlines what might happen if you don't have the operation, and what to expect when you are recovering from surgery.

The following pages provide general information on preparing for surgery, and what happens when you are taken to the operating theater. Each hospital, surgeon, anesthesiologist, and patient is different, however. This book can only provide general guidance. You need to obtain the specific information relating to your condition and your operation from your own healthcare providers. Never be afraid to ask questions — a good tip is to write down all the things you want to ask before your appointment, and to take the list with you. That way, you won't forget to obtain the important information you need during the stress of the moment.

I hope you find this book useful. Good luck!

PREPARING FOR SURGERY

If you are taking any medicines or supplements, tell your physician as some may affect blood clotting, or interfere with anesthetic drugs. It is especially important to tell your physician if you are taking aspirin or other medications, such as warfarin to thin your blood. The surgeon or anesthesiologist will tell you which medications you should stop taking and which you should continue to take before surgery.

The surgeon will fully explain the recommended procedure to you, along with the possible complications that can occur, the risks and benefits, and any alternative options. He or she will then usually ask you to sign a consent form to show that you understand the risks and agree to have the operation. This is known as informed consent.

When having an artificial implant, such as a hip or knee replacement, or a coronary artery bypass graft, you may be advised to have a dental evaluation beforehand. If you have significant dental disease (gingivitis, periodontitis), this may need to be treated before your operation to reduce the risk of mouth bacteria entering the circulation and infecting the new prosthesis.

> ## Pre-admission check list
> Think about whether you may need help with:
> • Cooking • Shopping • Bathing • Laundry
> • Gardening • Pet care • Transport

Loose teeth may also need to be removed in case they are dislodged and inhaled during insertion of the breathing tube during a general anesthetic.

You may be advised to donate some of your own blood prior to the surgery. It will then be stored in case you need to receive blood after your operation. This is the safest way to receive a blood transfusion as it cuts out the risk of a typing mis-match, and of acquiring a blood-borne infection. In the meantime, your body will make up the blood that was removed so that you are back to a normal level before your operation.

Try to be as fit and healthy as your condition allows before surgery. Try to lose at least some excess weight. If you smoke, do your utmost to stop. Smoking cigarettes increases the risk of abnormal blood clots, interferes with the healing process and lowers immunity to increase the risk of post-operative infections.

Although you may be able to walk unaided after surgery, you may be relatively immobile or need to rely on crutches. If you live alone, you need to think about how you will cope after going home, as you may need help with household tasks *(see page 10)*. You may also want to consider arranging a short stay in a convalescent facility during your recovery.

Think about whether you want to provide specific instructions for healthcare treatment in the event that you are unable to make or communicate these decisions personally after the operation. Known as an advanced directive, these can include a living will and durable power of attorney for health care. Advanced directives are legal documents and are displayed prominently in your medical records.

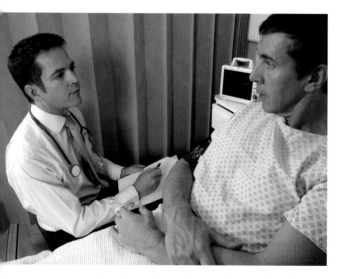

ABOVE A doctor on his ward round sits and talks with a male patient at his hospital bedside.

Before the operation

The anesthesiologist will discuss the type of anesthetic and post-operative pain relief you will receive. If having a general anesthetic, you will typically be asked not to eat or drink for about six hours (or overnight) before the operation. If you do, your operation may have to be canceled. Depending on the procedure, you may be allowed occasional sips of water for up to two hours beforehand.

If you have diabetes, the anesthesiologist will want to ensure your blood glucose levels are tightly controlled before, during, and after surgery. This helps to reduce the risk of infections, kidney problems, and other surgical complications. If your blood glucose levels are high (which can occur as a result of the stress associated with illness or having an operation), surgery may be postponed, unless absolutely essential, until your blood glucose control is acceptable.

You may have a chest X-ray, heart-tracing electrocardiogram (ECG or EKG), and blood tests before the operation to ensure that you are fit enough for surgery.

You may be asked to have a bath or shower before surgery.

Routine observations (blood pressure, pulse, temperature, respiratory rate) will be checked as a base line against which to assess post-operative findings. Your urine may be analyzed, too.

You will usually receive a pre-medication (pre-med) one or two hours before going to the operating theater. This is a drug to reduce anxiety, help you relax, and lower blood pressure. It may also include medication to reduce stomach acidity, dry up saliva, and reduce nausea.

You may be shaved to remove excess hair.

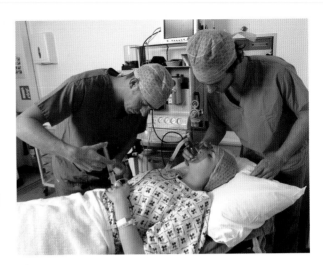

ABOVE An anesthesiologist administers anesthetic gases and drugs to put a patient to sleep at the start of an operation.

You will be asked to remove all jewelry, and any rings that cannot be taken off will be taped up so they do not get caught, or interfere with electrical cutting devices (diathermy).

You may be asked to put on graduated compression stockings to reduce the risk of a deep vein thrombosis or blood clot (DVT).

Local anesthesia

Many procedures are performed under local anesthesia as this is safer than a general anesthetic. This may involve:

Topical anesthesia — local anesthetic drops or gel are applied to the skin, eye, mouth, nose, airway, or urethra (urinary tube).

Local injections — anesthetic drugs are infiltrated into the skin and tissues around the operation site.

Field block — a more extensive area around the operation site is numbed to produce a pain-free zone.

Peripheral nerve block — an individual nerve supplying feeling to a small part of the body (e.g. hand, forearm) is numbed by injecting local anesthetic around the nerve at its root or along its course.

Regional block — a large nerve or nerve trunk supplying feeling to a region of the body (e.g. entire arm) is numbed by injecting local anesthetic around the nerve at its root.

Inform your surgeon

Always let your surgeon know about any previous medical conditions, operations, and general anesthetics you may have experienced. If you know you have a blood-borne infection, such as hepatitis B, hepatitis C, or HIV, always tell your healthcare providers.

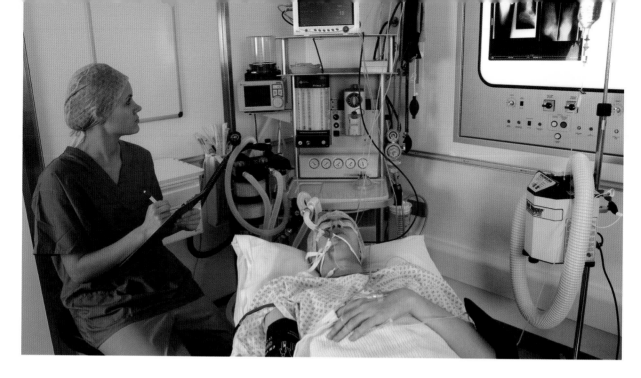

ABOVE A female anesthesiologist monitors a patient's condition during an operation.

Regional intravenous anesthesia — local anesthetic is injected into the veins of a limb that has had the blood squeezed out by wrapping it around with a tourniquet. This is a useful technique for hand operations *(see page 44, carpal tunnel release)*.

Spinal anesthesia — local anesthetic and analgesic drugs are injected directly into the subarachnoid space around the spinal cord to numb a large part of the body (for example, from the nipples downward).

Epidural anesthesia — local anesthetic and analgesic drugs are injected into the epidural space surrounding the spinal cord (this requires four to ten times more anesthetic drug than used in a spinal as it diffuses over a larger distance). Combined spinal-epidural anesthesia *(see page 20, cesarean section)* are increasingly popular as they provide rapid onset of numbness and excellent post-operative pain relief that can be topped up when necessary.

Allergic reactions

If you are allergic to iodine or any drugs, sticking plaster, or dressings, let your surgeon know before your operation.

General anesthesia

Before putting you to sleep, the anesthesiologist will insert a cannula into a vein in the back of your hand or side of your lower arm through which fluids and drugs can be injected. This is a little uncomfortable but most people can tolerate it without flinching.

A drug is injected into the cannula to put you to sleep, usually within ten to 20 seconds, or you may inhale an anesthetic gas plus oxygen through a mask. This usually takes place in a special side-room leading into the operating theater. The drugs and anesthetic gas mixture will be delivered continuously throughout the operation to maintain unconsciousness, and to relax and paralyze your muscles.

Once you are asleep, you are intubated, which means a breathing tube is placed directly into your windpipe (trachea) by passing it between your vocal cords. This allows careful administration of the correct mix of oxygen and anesthetic gas, which are pumped into your lungs using artificial ventilation as your breathing muscles are also paralyzed. You are attached to heart, blood pressure, pulse, and oxygen monitoring equipment that continuously assesses your vital signs. An intermittent pneumatic compression device may be used to compress your calves during surgery. This helps move blood through your deep leg veins to reduce the risk of a DVT.

During the operation

While the surgeon and assistant(s) scrub up (meaning that they wash and disinfect their hands and lower arms and don sterile surgical gowns and gloves), you will be lain on the operating table in the correct position. Sterile drapes will be placed over your body so that just the part of your body to be operated on is exposed.

You may have a catheter inserted into your bladder to drain away any residual urine. This may be a quick in-and-out procedure, or the catheter may be left in place for the duration of a major operation.

The surgeon cleanses the skin around the operating site with a strong antiseptic, such as povidone-iodine.

Before the surgeon closes the incision once the operation has been completed, the number of sponges, needles, and gauze swabs used are carefully counted to ensure that all are present, and that none has been left in the surgical cavity.

You are usually given some preventive drugs during or at the end of surgery. These may include: Prophylactic antibiotics, an antiemetic (to stop you being sick), antacids (to reduce the risk of peptic ulcers and inhalation of stomach acids), analgesics to reduce post-operative pain.

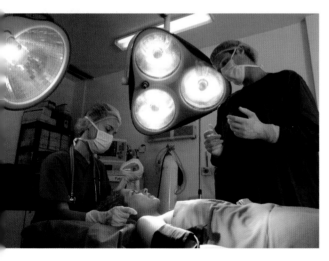

ABOVE A female anesthesiologist and male surgeon prepare a female patient at the start of an operation.

When you wake up

When you wake up, you may be aware of:
- An oxygen mask.
- A drip connected to a vein in your arm through which drugs and fluids are administered until you can start drinking properly.
- A blood pressure cuff around your arm which may inflate automatically from time to time.
- An oxygen monitor clipped to your fingertip (pulse oximeter).
- Dressings over your wound.
- Drain(s) collecting excess blood from the site of surgery.

After the operation

You will be closely observed by nursing staff immediately after the operation, while you come round from a general anesthetic.

Your blood pressure, pulse, respiratory rate, and temperature will be monitored and recorded regularly. The wound dressings will be checked and the amount of fluid draining from the wound site or catheter will be noted.

Don't be too concerned if you can't immediately move or feel part of your body, as it can take a while for the anesthetic to wear off, especially if you have received an epidural, spinal, or other type of nerve block.

It is important that you receive regular, adequate pain relief. Let the nursing staff know if you are in pain, as they can vary your dosage, change your analgesic medication, and give anti-sickness drugs if necessary.

If you are provided with patient controlled analgesia (PCA), you will be given a button which, when pressed firmly for a few seconds, delivers a dose of analgesic. Don't be afraid to use this regularly, exactly as advised, as it is easier to keep pain at bay than to get on top of it once it returns.

If you feel sick or dizzy, try taking a few deep breaths as oxygen can help to reduce these feelings. If they do not go away, tell the nursing staff.

You may be advised to perform deep breathing exercises to help clear your lungs and reduce the risk of a chest infection.

You can usually go home once you have recovered enough to be comfortable (using oral painkillers), to walk short distances on the flat, able to manage stairs (if appropriate), and any necessary help is in place at home.

After going home

Your surgeon will tell you how to care for your wound as it heals. In general, it is best to keep the area clean and dry. A dressing will be applied in the hospital and, if necessary, you will be given additional dressings and told how often they should be changed at home.

Do not shower or bathe until you are told that you can. Usually, this is once all sutures or staples have been removed, seven to ten days after surgery. Again, the wound should be kept clean and dry.

Let your physician know if the wound appears red, excessively painful, or begins to bleed, smell unpleasant, or drain pus.

Take your temperature twice a day and let your physician know if it rises above 100.5 °F (38 °C).

Seek immediate medical advice if you develop a painful or swollen calf, chest pain, or shortness of breath as these are signs of a possible blood clot.

Possible complications of surgery

Bleeding can occur after an operation. If this is going to happy, it usually occurs within the first few hours after surgery when blood vessels that have shut down as a result of being handled start to open up again. You will have your blood

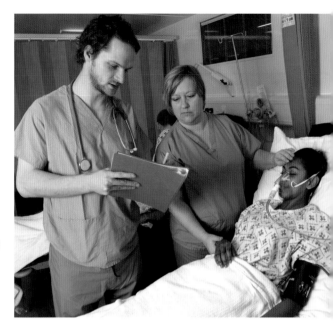

ABOVE A doctor and a nurse on their ward rounds check the condition of a woman patient wearing an oxygen mask.

pressure, pulse, and blood staining of dressings monitored regularly after a major operation so that this complication is diagnosed and treated promptly. In some cases, this may mean returning to surgery.

Swelling can occur, especially if a dressing or bandage is too tight, or if there is bleeding. This can reduce blood circulation and may interfere with breathing following a thyroid operation, for example. You will have your dressings and the color of your peripheries monitored regularly after a major operation to ensure that this complication is diagnosed and the dressing loosened promptly.

Infection can occur within the wound, within a body cavity (abscess), or in the bladder if a catheter is left in place. Prophylactic antibiotics are usually given during the operation to help reduce these complications, and may be continued afterward. Drains may also be inserted to remove any fluid or blood so there is no build-up to attract infection.

Chest infection can occur if you are immobilized and breathe shallowly due to pain. Adequate pain relief, early mobilization, and breathing exercises help to reduce this risk.

Leaving hospital

Before going home you are usually provided with:

• Any necessary medicines.

• A follow-up appointment.

• Instructions on how any clips or stitches will be removed.

• Spare dressings and instructions on how to change them, if necessary.

• Advice on any diet or exercises needed.

Septicemia (blood poisoning) can occur if bacteria enter the circulation (for example from a wound infection, or perforated bowel) and start to grow, producing toxins that can cause dramatic circulatory collapse (toxic shock).

Blood clots can develop, especially in the deep veins of the legs (deep vein thrombosis or DVT). These result from the increased stickiness of blood that develops after a major operation as part of the body's own wound healing response. Immobility and sometimes dehydration increase this risk, too. A part of the blood clot can break off and travel in the circulation to the lungs (pulmonary embolism) to affect breathing. To help prevent this, you may be asked to wear graduated compression stockings during and after the operation. A pneumatic device that compresses your calves during surgery may also be used to help stop blood pooling in the deep veins of your legs. The blood thinning agent, heparin, may also be injected just beneath your skin.

Keloids (excessive growth of scar tissue) can develop when an excessive healing response causes the formation of a thick scar. This tendency is most common over the sternum and shoulders. Unfortunately, attempts to remove a keloid with plastic surgery often result in new keloid formation. Fortunately, the appearance of most keloid scars can be improved by applying an adhesive, silicone gel sheet that flattens, softens, and fades red and raised scars.

Adhesions can develop as a result of the normal healing process within the abdominal and pelvic cavities. These strands of fibrous scar tissue start to form three to five days after surgery, and may cause internal organs to stick together. While they often cause no symptoms, they can cause

pain several months or even years after they originally formed *(see page 132)*.

Incisional hernias can form when an internal part of the body pushes through the weakness of a scar to form an external bulge. In extreme cases, these can be very large.

Possible complications of general anesthesia

Although rare, having a general anesthetic is associated with certain known risks including the precipitation of:

• Heart rhythm abnormalities.
• Angina.
• Heart attack.
• Congestive heart failure (fluid build-up in the lungs or lower body due to poor heart pumping).
• Stroke.
• Seizure.
• Allergic drug reactions.
• Asthma.
• Aspiration of stomach fluids which can lead to aspiration pneumonia.
• Collapsed lung (pneumothorax).
• Pulmonary embolism (blood clot in the lungs).
• Acute kidney failure.
• High fever (hyperthermia).
• Delirium.

The risk of death as a result of general anesthesia is very low at around one per 200,000 procedures, some of which are due to human error or equipment failure.

Cataract Extraction

Cataract extraction is the removal of the lens from one eye because it has developed a hardened opacity. This opacity, called a cataract, interferes with vision to cause cloudiness, increased glare, and decreased visual acuity. Usually, the lens is replaced with an artificial intraocular lens, which remains permanently inside the eye, to restore sight.

What causes cataracts?

Cataracts become increasingly common with age and most people over 65 have some degree of lens cloudiness. Known as senile cataract, this is linked with a lifetime's accumulation of free radical damage. Free radicals are molecular fragments that carry a minute negative charge. To achieve electrical stability, they pass on this negative charge through a process known as oxidation. This triggers damaging chain reactions in which electrical charges are passed from one atom to another at rapid speed. When this occurs within the eye lens, clear proteins may be oxidized to produce areas of cloudiness.

What causes free radicals?

Free radicals are produced continuously as a result of normal metabolism, but are generated in higher amounts in people with certain conditions, such as diabetes. Having poorly controlled diabetes can accelerate cataract formation so they develop ten to 15 years earlier than usual. Free radicals are also generated in higher amounts in people who smoke, drink excessive amounts of alcohol, and in those exposed to environmental pollutants, X-rays, UVA sunlight, and the use of certain medicines.

Free radical damage may be minimized by consuming plenty of antioxidant-rich fruit and vegetables. Antioxidants help to absorb and neutralize the negative charge on free radicals to reduce the damage they cause.

Why the lens is vulnerable

In order to transmit light without scatter, the lens does not contain any blood vessels, and is made of cells that lack a nucleus. Cells within the lens must therefore obtain their oxygen and nutrients by diffusion from the eye fluids in which the lens is suspended. This leaves the lens increasingly vulnerable to free radical attack when levels of antioxidant

CATARACT EXTRACTION AT A GLANCE

• *Can it be done as an outpatient?* Yes. Very few are performed as an inpatient.

• *Do I need a general anesthetic?* Not usually.

• *What special tests are needed?* Visual acuity is assessed for both near and far distances. A Type I cataract means visual acuity is better than 20/40 in the affected eye(s). A Type II cataract means that visual acuity is 20/40 or worse in the affected eye(s). Drops are instilled to dilate your pupils, so the back of your eye (retina, optic nerve, macula) is more easily examined. Eyes are also examined using a slit lamp and tonometry (which measures eye pressure). Before surgery, the correct power for your new intraocular lens is selected by measuring the curve of the front surface of your cornea (keratometry) and the size of your eye (biometry, using ultrasound).

• *How long does the surgery take?* Around 20 to 30 minutes.

• *What is the mortality rate?* Extremely low at less than one in 1000.

• *How long will I be in hospital?* Patients having the procedure as an inpatient usually stay for an average of four days.

• *How expensive is it?* 💲

• *How many are performed in the US each year?* Cataract procedures are among the most common surgical operations. An astonishing 3.1 million lens extractions for cataract are performed annually as an outpatient procedure, with 2.6 million prosthetic lenses inserted. In addition, around 1000 cataract procedures are performed as an inpatient. Just over 60% of patients are female, and the majority of patients are aged 65 and over.

nutrients are poor. Some evidence suggests that people with high dietary intakes of antioxidants (e.g. vitamins C, E, selenium, carotenoids) are less likely to develop cataracts *(for more information on prevention, see page 19).*

WHY AGE-RELATED LONGSIGHTEDNESS OCCURS

When light passes through the lens, it is focused upside-down onto the retina. Focusing is dependent upon the ability of the lens to change shape. At rest, the lens takes up a shape that is thin, flat, and naturally set up for distant vision. To focus on close objects, the lens becomes thicker, more convex, and its ability to refract light increases. The lens becomes less flexible with age, progressively losing its ability to focus light from near objects onto the retina. Known as presbyopia, this results in the onset of long vision which is usually noticed around the age of 45. By the age of 65, little close focusing ability remains, so that small print must be read at arm's length. Cataracts in older people are almost always accompanied by presbyopia, and replacing the eye lens with a prosthetic lens can significantly improve both problems.

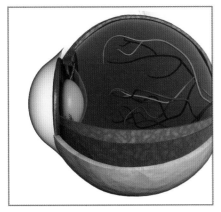

ABOVE Diagram showing a cross-section through an eye.

People without cataracts may also have a clear lens removed and replaced with an artificial one to correct severe long or short sightedness. This is known as CLEAR (Clear Lens Extraction and Replacement) surgery.

CATARACT EXTRACTION
STEP-BY-STEP

SELECTING THE RIGHT PROCEDURE

The management of cataracts is designed to correct visual impairment, maintain or improve quality of life, and to prevent the progression of lens cloudiness. Removal of the diseased lens and replacing it with an artificial intraocular lens is the treatment of choice. If both eyes are affected, they are usually operated on separately as this reduces the risk of a complication, such as infection, affecting vision in both eyes at the same time.

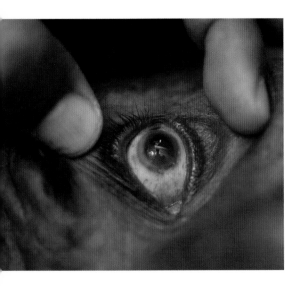

ABOVE **A patient with a cataract that requires extraction.**

Within the eye, the lens is contained within a clear, elastic, bag-like structure called the capsule. The capsule is attached to strong, suspensory ligaments that hold the lens in place in front of the pupil. During traditional cataract surgery, the entire lens was removed, together with its capsule — this is known as intracapsular cataract extraction (ICCE). It is now rarely performed.

ICCE has been replaced by extracapsular cataract extraction (ECCE) in which the lens is removed through a small opening in the front of the capsule. This leaves the posterior part of the capsule in place as a convenient "bag" into which a new lens may be inserted. This, in turn, has now been largely superseded by a third surgical option called phacoemulsification, or phaco for short (from the Greek word, phakos, meaning lens). Phaco is similar to ECCE, in that the lens is removed through an opening in the capsule, which is left behind. Rather than manual removal of the lens, however, it is fragmented using ultrasound and removed by sucking it out through a needle.

Phacoemulsification or ECCE are used wherever possible as they involve smaller incisions than ICCE, less risk of complications, more rapid wound healing, and faster return of acceptable vision. Phaco is the treatment of choice as only a tiny wound is produced that often does not need sutures. As the wound is so small, a foldable artificial

Alpha-blocker drugs and cataract surgery

Alpha-blocker drugs are widely used to treat high blood pressure, and to improve urinary symptoms in both women and men. They are especially used to treat male symptoms associated with an enlarged prostate gland. People taking an alpha-blocker drug may experience a complication during cataract surgery known as intraoperative floppy iris syndrome. As well as relaxing muscles in the prostate gland, these drugs can cause muscles in the iris to constrict suddenly during cataract surgery. This may mean the operation cannot be completed. Almost all (95%) of 1000 surgeons responding to a survey by the American Society of Cataract and Refractive Surgery, in 2008, said that they had encountered intraoperative floppy iris syndrome while performing cataract extraction. Always tell your doctor which drugs you are taking before undergoing surgery.

lens is rolled up and inserted with phaco, while a non-foldable lens is replaced through the larger incision produced during ECCE.

During surgery, you will lie on an operating table or sit back in a reclining chair. Your eyelid is swabbed with antiseptic solution and your face covered with a sterile cloth that has an eye-shaped opening through which the surgeon operates.

❶ Eye drops are instilled 30 to 60 minutes before surgery to constrict blood vessels (which reduces bleeding) and to maximally dilate the iris (colored part of the eye). This produces a wide pupil which makes removal of the lens easier.

❷ Sedation is usually given (orally or into a vein) to reduce anxiety and may mean that you remember little of the procedure afterward. A local anesthetic gel is instilled to numb the front of the eye. Local anesthetic may also be injected next to and behind the eyeball. The eyelids are then held open with a speculum to stop you blinking *(see page 16)*. Artificial tears are used to keep the front of the eye moist.

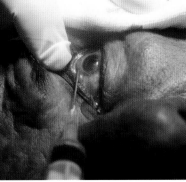

ABOVE A surgeon injects local anesthetic to numb the eye.

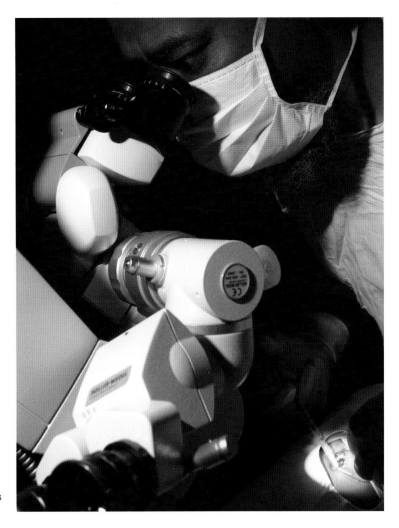

RIGHT A surgeon operates using a binocular instrument that gives him a magnified view of the eye.

REMOVING THE LENS

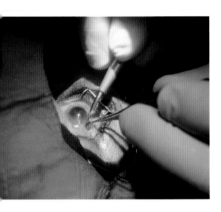

ABOVE A surgeon makes an incision into the limbus (where the cornea meets the sclera).

BELOW A surgeon uses an ultrasound probe (top) and chopper (bottom) to break up a cataract. The resulting fragments are sucked away.

❸ The surgeon makes a small incision near where the cornea meets the white of the eye (sclera) *(see left)*. A thick (viscoelastic) gel may be injected to help maintain pressure in the front of the eye and stabilize the iris. Instruments are then inserted to make a small, round, smooth hole in the front of the lens capsule. If performing ECCE, a larger hole is needed to remove the lens manually. For phaco, only a small hole is needed through which the ultrasonic probe is inserted. This has a fine, needle tip that vibrates at a frequency of 40,000 times per second, transmitting energy to the lens to break it up.

❹ The ultrasound needle is used to sculpt trenches across the cataract, sucking up the emulsified fragments. A second ultrasound tool (known as a chopper) may be held in the other hand to help crack the hardened cataract into two to four smaller pieces which are then emulsified and sucked away *(see below)*. This is known as the "divide and conquer" technique. The softer, outer parts of the lens are removed with suction only, to leave behind an empty lens capsule.

❺ An artificial lens is now inserted into the empty lens capsule. Foldable lenses (made from silicone or acrylic) can be inserted, using a special introducer, through incisions that are less than 0.12 in (3 mm) across. A non-foldable intraocular lens (made from polymethylacrylate) requires a larger incision and may be inserted following ECCE.

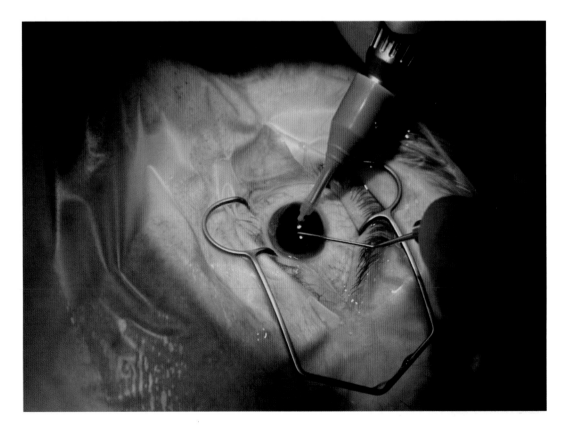

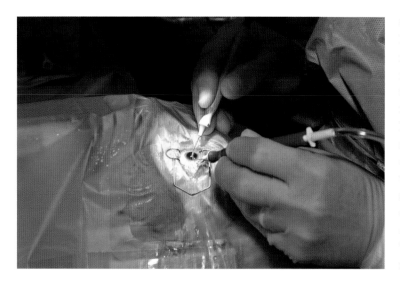

❻ After inserting the artificial lens *(see left)*, the surgeon removes the viscoelastic material injected into the front of the eye, and checks that the small incision in the cornea has self-sealed. If it leaks fluid, a temporary nylon suture may be needed to stitch it closed. The knot is rotated into the cornea to reduce irritation, and the suture is removed after one week. Antibiotic and steroid drops are applied, and a clear "bandage" contact lens or patch may be used to cover the eye.

ABOVE A surgeon uses probes to place an artificial intraocular lens implant into the lens capsule.

RIGHT AND BELOW An intraocular lens implant is monitored on screen as it is carefully moved into position by the surgeon.

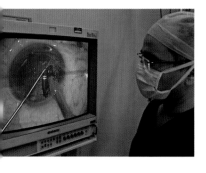

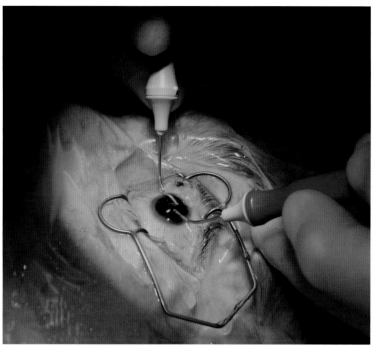

Artificial lenses

Originally, single-power, fixed-focus artificial lenses were implanted that allowed you to see far distances, but required additional glasses for near vision. Modern multifocal and adaptive (accommodating) intraocular lenses mean you can usually see well through a variety of distances, but these are significantly more expensive. Some surgeons recommend a "mix and match" approach in which a multifocal lens is inserted in one eye for close reading, while an accommodating lens is placed in the other eye for midrange vision. Intraocular lenses are made of flexible plastic and have side struts that hold them in place within the lens capsule. Accommodating lenses are designed to move back and forth as the focusing muscles attached to the lens capsule constrict or relax.

Cataract Extraction
Questions & Answers

What are the benefits?

Cataract extraction and intraocular lens replacement can improve vision in 95% of patients. In those whose vision is not restored, other conditions may be present such as age-related macular degeneration (AMD) or diabetic retinopathy.

What are the risks?

As well as the general risks associated with surgery and general anesthesia *(see pages 10–11)*, you may experience some visual disturbances. Usually vision is clear after cataract surgery, but one in five people experience cloudiness or blurred vision as a result of a posterior capsule opacity which develops a year or so after surgery. This is easily treated, painlessly, by using a YAG laser to make a hole in the hazy part of the capsule (capsulotomy) so it no longer interferes with your line of sight. This procedure takes only a few minutes and is performed after dilation of your pupil with drops. You may experience a few "floaters" after the procedure, but these usually resolve within a few weeks. Other complications of cataract surgery include loosening or dislocation of the new intraocular lens, experiencing "halos" around lights at nighttime, and developing eye inflammation, eye infections, or increased pressure in the eye (glaucoma). Complications of surgery may result in irreversible blindness in one eye in around 1% of cases.

Are there any alternatives?

Eye glasses may improve visual acuity. Researchers are investigating whether or not a type of drug called an aldose reductase inhibitor, which reduces the conversion of glucose to sorbitol within cells, may reduce the progression of cataracts in people with diabetes. Cataracts may improve in people taking vitamin C tablets (n.b. vitamin C can affect blood and urine tests used to assess glucose control in diabetes — check with your doctor before taking them).

What can I do to prepare?

Try to ensure that you are as fit as possible. If you smoke, do your utmost to stop, as smoking increases the risk of infection and impairs healing. You may be asked to start using eye drops containing a non-steroidal anti-inflammatory drug (e.g. nepafenac) the day before surgery. Ask your surgeon about taking vitamin C tablets, which may help to reduce inflammation after surgery and promote healing of the cornea.

What if I don't have the operation?

Vision is likely to continue deteriorating. An untreated cataract can result in lens swelling, glaucoma (increased pressure within the eye), and eventual blindness.

What happens during the recovery period?

The drops instilled into the eye before surgery continue to work for three to five hours, so vision is blurred initially.

Corticosteroid eye drops (e.g. prednisolone, dexamethasone) help to reduce inflammation and swelling after surgery. These are usually combined with antibiotics which are used for one to two weeks after eye surgery to help prevent infection.

Eye drops containing a non-steroidal anti-inflammatory drug (e.g. nepafenac) may be used to reduce pain and swelling, starting one day before surgery and continuing for two weeks afterward.

It takes two to three weeks to recover fully from cataract surgery. During this time, avoid strenuous exercise and anything that might cause a rise in blood pressure.

You will have regular eye checks after surgery and may require glasses to achieve optimum corrected vision.

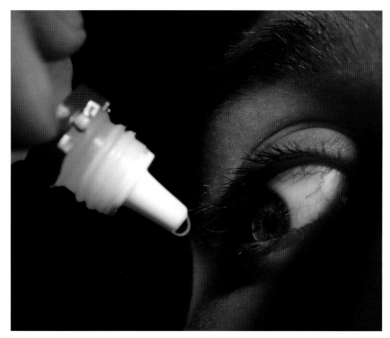

RIGHT Applying treatment drops to the eye. After cataract surgery, eye drops are prescribed to reduce inflammation and swelling, and control pain.

Lifestyle modifications

- Research suggests that following a diet rich in antioxidants may reduce the development and delay the progression of cataracts. Vegetables such as spinach, broccoli, and carrots, which contain carotenoid plant pigments, are especially beneficial.
- Wearing sunglasses helps to protect the eyes from ultraviolet rays. Select those that block 99% or 100% of all UV light (n.b. "UV absorption up to 400 nm" is the same as 100% protection). Sunglasses that are close fitting or wrap-around help to prevent light entering your eyes around the frame of the glasses.

CESAREAN SECTION

A cesarean section — often referred to as a C-section or just a section — is the surgical delivery of a baby through an incision made in the mother's abdomen. A cesarean section may be carried out on a planned date, as an elective procedure, or in an emergency when the well-being of the mother or baby is at risk.

ELECTIVE CESAREAN

An elective cesarean is performed when a normal vaginal delivery is likely to cause unnecessary risk to the health, or life, of either mother or baby. In some cases, having an elective cesarean is a lifestyle choice for mothers wishing to fit the delivery into their busy schedule, or because they do not wish to experience a normal vaginal birth.

An obstetrician may suggest that you have an elective cesarean for a number of reasons, not all of which make the operation essential. The final decision about whether to have an elective cesarean, or a trial of labor (to see if you can successfully deliver normally), is only made after carefully weighing up the pros and cons with both you and, where appropriate, your partner. Common indications for an elective cesarean include multiple pregnancy (twins or more), breech position (in which the baby is head up rather than head down), and medical conditions that increase the risk of normal delivery for you (e.g. high blood pressure, heart problems) or your baby (e.g. fetal abnormalities, HIV infection, primary genital herpes infection). You are also more likely to have an elective cesarean if you are over the age of 40 (when complications such as failure to progress are more likely) or if you have previously had a cesarean section.

An elective cesarean is usually planned for the 39th week of pregnancy, so the baby's lungs

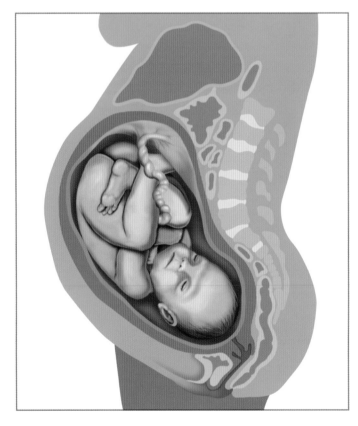

BELOW At 37–42 weeks a baby is considered full term and usually measures approximately 19.5 in (50 cm) from the head to the heel. It normally weighs around 7 lb (3 kg).

CESAREAN SECTION AT A GLANCE

- *Can it be done as an outpatient?* No. Admission to hospital is necessary.

- *Do I need a general anesthetic?* A general anesthetic may be needed in an emergency where rapid delivery is essential. When time allows, the preferred method is either an epidural or a combined spinal and epidural *(see page 8).* An epidural injects local anesthetic into the epidural space outside the membranes surrounding your spinal cord. In combined spinal-epidural anesthesia, a local anesthetic is also injected beneath the membranes, into the cerebrospinal fluid bathing your spinal cord. This lets you remain awake so that you can see your baby immediately after birth. The epidural can provide post-operative pain relief too.

- *What special tests are needed?* Before an elective cesarean, ultrasound scans help to assess a baby's growth, development, breathing movements, and muscle tone. Before an emergency cesarean, the baby's heartbeat and your contractions are assessed using an external fetal monitor strapped to your abdomen. Internal monitoring may be used when the cervical canal is dilated enough to allow insertion of a pressure catheter and a fetal scalp electrode.

- *How long does the surgery take?* An emergency cesarean can deliver the baby within two minutes. In a more relaxed elective cesarean, the baby is usually delivered within ten minutes. In both cases, it then takes another 30 to 45 minutes to deliver the placenta (afterbirth), control bleeding, and sew the wound. The operation can take longer if scar tissue is present from previous cesareans.

- *What is the mortality rate?* The maternal mortality rate is very low at less than 0.01% (one death per 10,000 procedures).

- *How long will I be in hospital?* Three to four days.

- *How expensive is it?* 💲

- *How many are performed in the US each year?* Around 1,350,000 cesarean sections are carried out per year, representing around one in three births. There is a trend toward the number of cesareans to increase year by year.

are as mature as possible before birth. This reduces the risk of respiratory distress which can develop if the infant is delivered too early. Earlier delivery may be needed, however, for example in the case of multiple births or where pregnancy is complicated by diabetes, high blood pressure, or if the baby is not growing properly (intrauterine growth retardation).

EMERGENCY CESAREAN

An emergency cesarean is performed after labor has started, when complications develop that put the well-being of mother or baby at risk. It is often needed when labor fails to progress, especially where the baby is large and the mother is exhausted or delivery using forceps or suction (ventouse) is unsuccessful. An emergency section is also needed when a baby shows severe signs of distress during monitoring, such as increased or decreased heart rate, during or after a contraction. Other indications include umbilical cord compression or prolapse (where the cord is delivered first, which reduces blood supply if the baby follows through the birth canal) and placental complications such as placenta previa (in which the placenta covers the cervical canal) or abruption (early separation of the placenta).

CESAREAN SECTION
STEP-BY-STEP

LOWER SEGMENT CESAREAN SECTION

The traditional cesarean involved a laparotomy up-and-down midline incision *(see page 132)* but this is rarely used today. The most common procedure is a lower segment cesarean section (LSCS) in which a transverse cut is made along the bikini line. Unless the procedure is a dire emergency, your birth partner is usually able to attend the operation to support you and share the experience. Drapes are carefully arranged over a frame so neither you nor your partner can see the actual surgery, but you can see the baby as he or she is lifted into the air. Usually you will receive an epidural or combined epidural and spinal anesthesia *(see page 25)* before being wheeled into the operating theater. You may have an oxygen mask placed over your nose and mouth to help increase the oxygen supply to your baby before delivery.

❶ The operating table is tilted slightly to the left, or you may have a pillow placed under your lower right back to prevent you lying fully on your back. This stops the uterus from pressing down on the large blood vessels (aorta, inferior vena cava) at the back of your abdomen, which can cause low blood pressure (supine hypotension syndrome). The surgeon then makes a horizontal incision along the lower abdomen, usually just below the pubic hair line. This is known as a Pfannenstiel or bikini incision. The wound is around 6 in (15 cm) long, and is made using a hot "knife" that seals (cauterizes) the tissues to reduce bleeding.

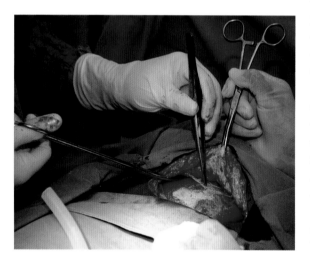

ABOVE The surgeon exposes the uterus through an incision in the lower abdominal wall.

❷ The surgeon carefully cuts through the skin and underlying layers of fat and connective tissue covering the two muscles (rectus abdominis) that run up and down the center of your abdomen *(see left)*. These muscles are separated and pulled apart (using fingers) without cutting, to expose the lower segment of the uterus. The surgeon picks up and cuts the fold of peritoneal membrane that runs between the uterus and bladder to expose the

Vertical incision

Sometimes a small up-and-down incision may be made that extends from just below the umbilicus (belly button) into the pubic hair just above the pubic bone. This allows more rapid extraction of the baby in an emergency. It is also indicated if a lot of scar tissue is present from previous cesarean sections, if the baby is lying crosswise (transverse), or if there are certain fetal abnormalities, such as conjoined twins.

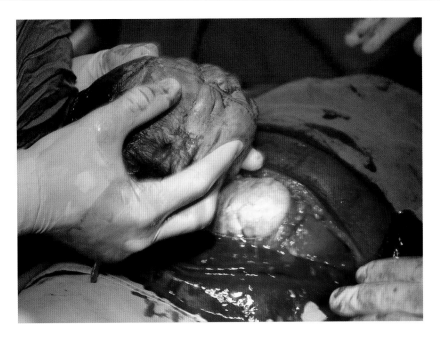

RIGHT When the baby is in the normal head-down position, the surgeon grasps the baby's head and carefully delivers it through the cesarean incision.

underlying uterine muscle. A bladder retractor is placed over the pubic bone to hold down the bladder and protect it from injury. An incision is then made into the muscular wall of the lower uterine segment and stretched open.

❸ The surgeon cuts into the amniotic membranes covering the baby. An assistant is ready with a tube to suck up the large gush of amniotic fluid that is released.

❹ The surgeon places one hand inside the uterine cavity, between the wall of the uterus and the baby's head. Using fingers, the surgeon gently lifts and guides the baby's head through the incision, taking care not to tear the incision wider *(see above)*. An assistant applies pressure to the top of the uterus (fundus) to help deliver the head. If the baby's head is deep down in the pelvis or vagina, as may happen after a prolonged labor, an assistant may need to push the baby's head up through the vagina before delivery through the incision can occur. The baby's shoulders and body are then delivered.

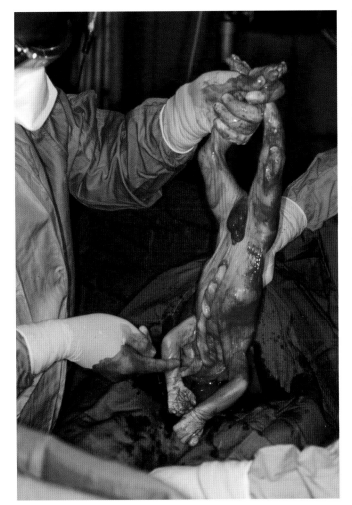

LEFT When the baby is in a breech position, the surgeon delivers the baby feet first through the cesarean incision.

Once the head is delivered, the baby's nose and mouth are gently sucked clear of fluid using a tiny tube. At this time, the anesthesiologist gives the mother an injection of the hormone-like drug oxytocin, which causes the uterus to contract. This aids delivery of the placenta.

❺ The umbilical cord is clamped *(see below)* and cut, and the baby is handed to an assistant for continued care. A dose of antibiotics is usually given to the mother at this stage to help prevent infection. The surgeon then pulls on the cord and gently rubs the top of the uterus through the abdominal wall to deliver the placenta and membranes.

❻ The uterus is closed using absorbable sutures — it is often pulled out through the incision for easier access, then tucked back inside. The abdominal cavity is flushed with saline to remove amniotic fluid and blood, and to check for any continued bleeding. The abdominal wound is then closed with absorbable sutures that dissolve over time, or with staples that are removed three to five days later.

BELOW **The umbilical cord is clamped before it is cut.**

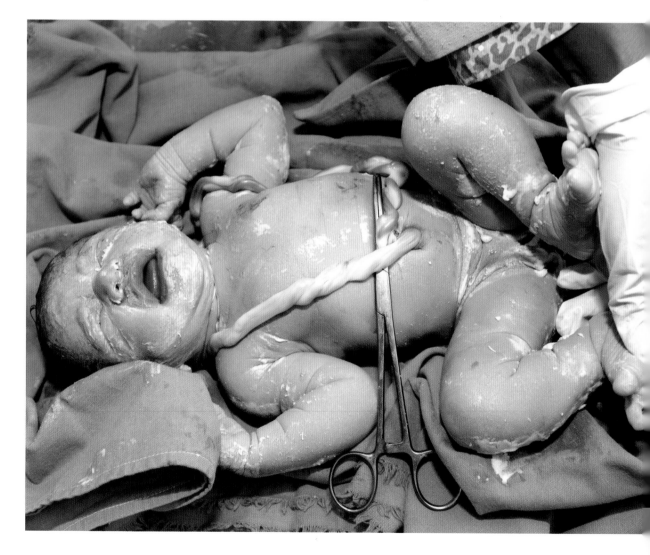

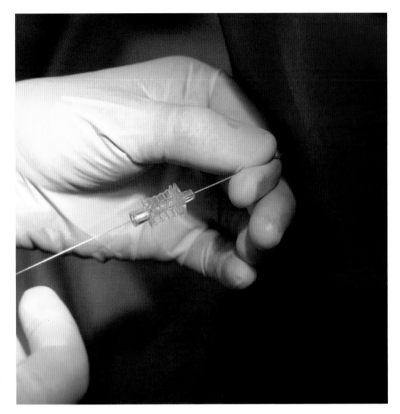

RIGHT An anesthesiologist inserts a guide needle into a catheter for an epidural.

Epidural and combined spinal and epidural anesthesia

- An intravenous drip is set up and your pulse and blood pressure are monitored.
- You will be asked to curve around your bump if lying on your side, or to curl forward over your bump if sitting up.
- The skin over your lower back is cleaned with antiseptic, then injected with a local anesthetic.
- An epidural needle is gently inserted between two of your lower back bones (lumbar vertebrae) until the anesthesiologist feels the loss of resistance as the needle enters the epidural space surrounding your spinal cord.
- If you are having a combined spinal and epidural, another needle is inserted through the first needle to puncture the underlying membrane (dura mater) and inject local anesthetic into the cerebrospinal fluid; this second needle is then removed.
- A small, flexible plastic tube (catheter) is threaded through the epidural needle into your epidural space. The epidural needle is then removed and the catheter taped to your back.
- Local anesthetic can now be injected through the catheter, into your epidural space, for continuous or top-up pain relief.

The spinal injection works almost instantly to remove all sensation and ability to move from the level of your nipples downward. Its effects wear off within 60 to 90 minutes, however. An epidural provides similar loss of sensation and pain but works more slowly — ten to 30 minutes to take effect. It can be topped up to provide pain relief for as long as necessary, however, and for post-op pain relief. Combining the techniques provides the benefits of both, making it a popular option for cesarean sections. An opiate painkiller is often injected along with the local anesthetic for improved analgesia. Although you will not feel any pain, you may feel some pulling and tugging movements, which should not hurt.

Cesarean Section
Questions & Answers

What are the benefits?

An emergency cesarean can be life-saving for both mother and child. Women who have had a cesarean are slightly less likely to develop future urinary stress incontinence than women who have delivered normally (16% versus 21%) but these findings should not be used to justify having an elective cesarean section.

What are the risks?

The risks associated with an elective "low risk" cesarean delivery (e.g. for breech presentation) are small, but are greater than those associated with normal vaginal delivery. There is a higher risk of infection (puerperal sepsis), blood clots (deep vein thrombosis, embolism), and heart attack, but, in general, the difference in the maternal mortality rate between an elective cesarean and a normal delivery is not significant. The risks associated with high risk pregnancies and emergency sections are obviously greater, however.

As well as the general risks associated with surgery and general anesthesia *(see pages 10–11)*, having a cesarean causes scarring of the womb which increases the chance of complications during a future delivery, including uterine rupture and abnormally deep attachment of the placenta (placenta accreta) which can hemorrhage during removal. Spinal or epidural anesthesia can cause severe headache that comes on hours to days afterward, as a result of cerebrospinal fluid leaking into the epidural space. This is treated with painkillers and bed rest. Occasionally a small amount of blood must be injected into the epidural space which clots to "patch" the leak.

Are there any alternatives?

In some cases an obstetrician who has recommended an elective cesarean may allow a "trial of labor" to see if you can deliver normally. This will depend on the reasons why surgery was originally suggested. Some obstetricians will support a woman wishing to have a vaginal birth following an LSCS in a previous pregnancy, as long as facilities are available to proceed to immediate emergency cesarean when necessary.

If labor is advanced, emergency cesarean can sometimes be avoided by using forceps or suction (ventouse) to extract the baby vaginally.

What can I do to prepare?

If you know you are having a cesarean, it is important to get into the right frame of mind. Some women feel they have somehow failed because they have lost control over the birthing process. Try to remain positive — having carried your baby and brought him or her safely into the world, it shouldn't really matter which route they used to arrive.

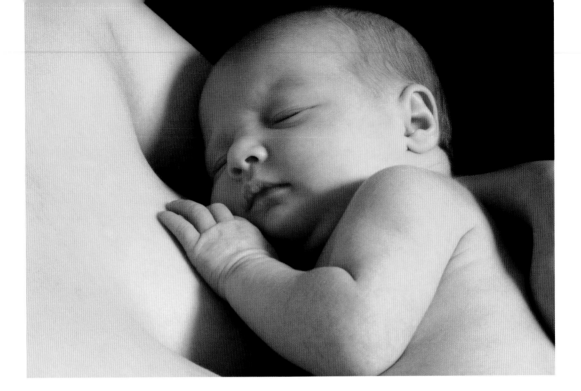

Think about whom you want to attend the cesarean birth — while this may be your partner, some women prefer to have their own mother, sister, or best friend supporting them instead. Some partners may feel too squeamish to attend, so it is important to discuss this openly.

You may find it helpful to attend a childbirth class that describes what happens during a cesarean section, and to visit a delivery suite and neonatal intensive care unit if your baby is likely to require specialist care.

What if I don't have the operation?

It is important to discuss the risks of not having the operation with your obstetrician. In some cases, a women who is advised to have an elective cesarean may still be able to have a successful vaginal delivery, as not all indications for surgery mean an operation is mandatory. However, not having a cesarean section may put the well-being of mother and/or baby at risk.

What happens during the recovery period?

Your baby will be brought to you as soon as possible, so you can put him or her to the breast, and start bonding with the new addition to your family. If your baby needs medical treatment in the neonatal intensive care unit, you will usually be given a photograph of him or her to keep with you until you are able to sit in a wheelchair and be taken to their side. You will be encouraged to mobilize within 24 hours. Pain relief is given as necessary. You may experience minor discomfort or, often, skin numbness around the cesarean scar for several months afterward. During future pregnancies your obstetrician will discuss with you the pros and cons of having another cesarean versus a normal vaginal birth.

CHOLECYSTECTOMY

Cholecystectomy is the surgical removal of the gallbladder (cholecyst). This pouch-like organ has only one function — to store bile, a green-yellow, detergent-like substance made in the liver. When you eat, the gallbladder contracts to squirt bile into your gut. Bile breaks down dietary fat into small globules (emulsification) which are easier to absorb. The gallbladder is usually removed because of symptoms associated with gallstones.

WHAT ARE GALLSTONES?

Gallstones are solid collections of material that can precipitate out of bile within the gallbladder. Most gallstones are made of cholesterol, although some contain large amounts of bile pigments or calcium salts. They tend to be round or oval in shape, and range in size from 0.04 in to 1 in (1 mm to 25 mm) across. Some people develop one large stone, while others harbor up to 200 or more small, grit-like stones.

Gallstones are three or four times more common in women than in men. They are especially common in women who have used the oral contraceptive pill or estrogen replacement therapy for two or more years.

WHAT ARE THE SYMPTOMS OF GALLSTONES?

Only one in five people with gallstones develops symptoms. Gallstones are often found by chance, when another condition is investigated, for example during computed tomographic (CT) scanning for other causes of abdominal pain. Those that stay in the gallbladder tend to remain "silent" — it's when they try to leave the gallbladder and pass into the sensitive bile duct that symptoms develop.

Gallstone pain usually begins suddenly, across the upper abdomen after a fatty meal. The pain is often difficult to locate exactly and may settle in the upper right part of the abdomen, or spread to between the shoulder blades or under the right shoulder. The pain is severe and tends to come and go in waves. This is known as biliary colic. Some people feel sick, or vomit, and belching is common. If the stone blocks the flow of bile, the person may become jaundiced.

Gallstones can lead to inflammation or infection of the gallbladder (acute cholecystitis) in which biliary pain is longer-lasting, there is abdominal tenderness, and fever. Research shows that having the gallbladder removed early during an episode of acute cholecystitis leads to earlier recovery and improved outcomes than the traditional approach of waiting for six weeks until inflammation has settled down.

CHOLECYSTECTOMY AT A GLANCE

• **Can it be done as an outpatient?** Yes (laparoscopically — *see page 30*).

• **Do I need a general anesthetic?** Yes.

• **What special tests are needed?** The diagnosis of biliary colic is usually confirmed using ultrasound scanning, which can detect 95% of all gallstones. It may miss very tiny stones and those lodged in the bile duct system. Ultrasound also shows thickening of the gallbladder wall if cholecystitis is present. If a gallstone is thought to be lodged in the bile duct, a special dye test called a cholangiogram is carried out, in which X-rays of the bile ducts are taken after injecting a special fluid that shows up on X-rays. The fluid may be injected into the blood stream to become concentrated in the bile and gallbladder. Alternatively, the "dye" may be injected via a fine catheter that is passed down through the mouth, stomach, and duodenum, and up into the bile duct (ERCP or endoscopic retrograde cholangiopancreatography). After the "dye" enters the bile ducts, any stones will show up on X-ray.

• **How long does the surgery take?** A laparoscopic cholecystectomy takes around an hour. An operation started laparoscopically, which is then converted to open cholecystectomy, may take from one and a half to three hours, as this usually occurs when a difficult situation, such as dense adhesions or unusual anatomy, are present. A mini-laparotomy cholecystectomy takes around 45 minutes. Cholangiography (X-ray during surgery to check for gallstones in the common bile duct) usually adds no more than five minutes to surgery time.

• **What is the mortality rate?** Less than one in a 100 (0.68%).

• **How long will I be in hospital?** Patients usually stay in hospital for an average of four to five days with an open operation. Those having a laparoscopic cholecystectomy can often go home the day after surgery if there are no complications.

• **How expensive is it?** 💲💲

• **How many are performed in the US each year?** Around 390,000 operations are performed as an inpatient in the US each year. In addition, around 500,000 laparoscopic cholecystectomies are performed on an outpatient basis. Two thirds of operations involve people aged 45 years or over. Two thirds of people having a cholecystectomy are female.

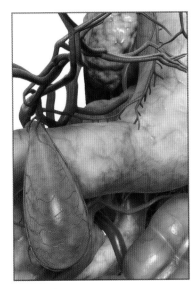

ABOVE Diagram of the stomach and gallbladder (bottom left).

There is an increased risk of bile duct injury during the operation, however.

If you develop biliary colic, you are usually advised to have a cholecystectomy as the severe pain is likely to recur. Gallstones not causing symptoms may be left alone, but are often removed electively to prevent future problems, especially in younger adults. Recent research suggests that having small gallstones may increase the risk of developing inflammation of the pancreas (pancreatitis). A rare reason for needing a cholecystectomy is because of gallbladder cancer.

Gallstones are linked with:
• Eating a fatty, high-cholesterol diet.
• Advancing age — up to one in ten older people have them.
• Taking the oral contraceptive pill or estrogen replacement therapy.
• A raised cholesterol level.
• Liver diseases that affect bile composition.

CHOLECYSTECTOMY STEP-BY-STEP

OPEN OR LAPAROSCOPIC CHOLECYSTECTOMY

The most popular way to remove the gallbladder is using keyhole surgery (laparoscopic cholecystectomy) which is attempted in 95% of cases. If difficulties are experienced or foreseen during laparoscopy, the surgeon will immediately convert to an open operation. This is not seen as a failure of surgical technique, but simply as safe practice. Conversion to an open operation occurs in less than 1% of operations for uncomplicated gallstones, rising to 5% of operations in which acute cholecystitis is present.

An open operation (mini-laparotomy cholecystectomy) is usually planned from the start for a patient who has previously undergone upper abdominal surgery. This is because adhesions and scar tissue are likely to cause problems identifying the correct anatomy. An open operation is also advised in people with known cirrhosis of the liver, in pregnant women, and where there is a suspected gallbladder or other cancer.

After being anesthetized, the patient is placed on a radiolucent operating table, through which X-rays can pass. This allows X-ray imaging (cholangiography) to be performed if necessary *(see page 32)*. A nasogastric tube is then passed down through the nose to deflate the stomach. This improves visibility during surgery, reduces the risk of accidental perforation, and also stops stomach acids being pushed up into the throat when air is pumped into the abdominal cavity to improve the view.

LAPAROSCOPIC CHOLECYSTECTOMY

BELOW Operating through a small incision *(see Mini-laparotomy box, page 31)*.

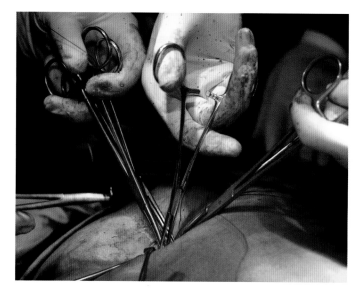

❶ An incision is made in the lower umbilicus (belly button) and air is pumped into the abdominal cavity *(see bottom image, opposite)*. The laparoscope (camera) is inserted through this incision and the abdominal and pelvic organs thoroughly examined to exclude any unforeseen problems. The operating table is then tilted slightly head up, and sideways toward the left, so the intestines fall away from the liver and gallbladder area. If, after inspecting the liver and gallbladder, the surgeon is happy to proceed laparoscopically, he does so.

❷ Three more small incisions are made in the abdominal wall, one to grasp the top of the gallbladder, one to manipulate the neck of the gallbladder, and one through which the main surgical cutting instruments are passed. One incision is usually in the midline just below the ribs, close to the gallbladder. The position of the remaining two incisions can vary from surgeon to surgeon. Some make two incisions in the lower right abdomen, while others prefer to make one incision to the lower right, and one to the lower left. If the liver has a floppy lobe that obstructs the surgeon's view of the gallbladder, an additional incision may be needed to insert a liver retractor.

❸ The pouch of the gallbladder is grasped with blunt forceps and pushed up over the liver, toward the diaphragm, as far as it will go. If it is very distended, it is punctured with a needle and syringe to suck out some of the contents (these are sent to the laboratory to look for signs of infection). Flimsy adhesions between the gallbladder and liver are pulled off using fine forceps. Thicker adhesions are carefully burned through and sealed using a hot knife (diathermy).

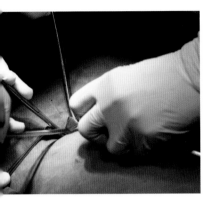

ABOVE The surgeon repositions retractors in preparation for the next stage during a mini-laparotomy cholecystectomy.

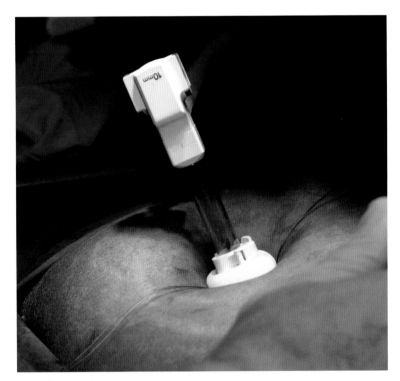

RIGHT Inserting the laparoscope.

Mini-laparotomy cholecystectomy

This open operation is performed through a small (2 in / 5 cm) incision in the right upper abdomen, beneath the ribs (see opposite and above left). Sometimes a longer incision (6 in / 15 cm) is needed to gain access. Retractors are used to hold back the sides of the wound. Moistened packs are inserted to retract and protect the liver and intestines. Calot's triangle is then explored, and the cystic artery and cystic duct sealed and cut before dissecting out the gallbladder and removing it. The packs are then removed and the abdomen closed in layers, as for a standard laparotomy incision (see page 136).

Identifying Calot's triangle

❹ Holding the neck of the gallbladder with another set of forceps, the surgeon then identifies an anatomical triangle between the common hepatic duct, the cystic duct (leading from the gallbladder to the common bile duct), and the liver. This is called Calot's triangle, and is important because it contains the cystic artery which supplies blood to the gallbladder. Tissue in this area is carefully dissected out until the cystic artery and the cystic duct are positively identified. If the cholangiogram is satisfactory, these two structures are each clipped and sealed using two titanium clips, absorbable clips, or a suture loop, depending on surgeon preference. If the cholangiogram shows a stone in the bile duct, it must be explored either laparoscopically, by converting to an open operation, or post-operatively through an endoscopic procedure that approaches through the intestinal end of the duct.

BELOW A minimally invasive cholecystectomy using a laparoscope and laser equipment.

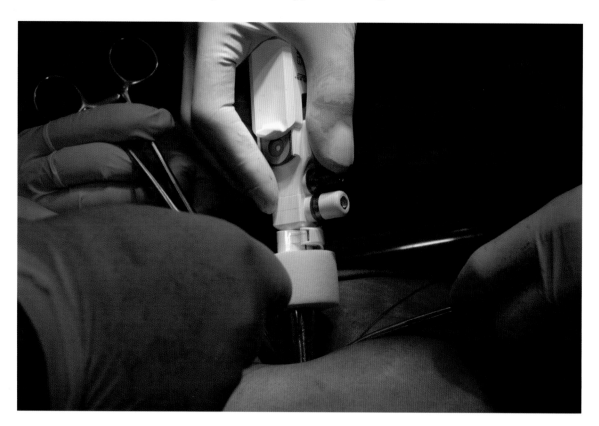

Cholangiography

Some surgeons perform a routine cholangiogram during a cholecystectomy to prove there are no gallstones lodged in the bile duct. Others only carry out this X-ray procedure if the patient has been jaundiced, if the common bile duct is dilated, or if liver blood tests are abnormal.

It is also helpful if someone has unusual bile duct anatomy with extra ducts present. Some hospitals use real-time fluoroscopic imagery which shows results immediately, without having to wait for X-ray films to be developed and returned.

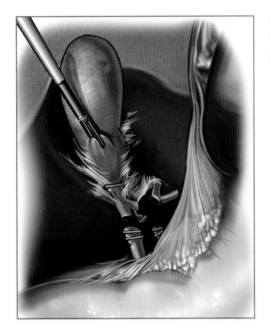

ABOVE The gallbladder being removed — the common bile duct has accidentally been cut and needs to be repaired.

❺ The gallbladder is now carefully dissected away from the liver using scissors or a hot knife *(see left)*. Some people have an additional small bile duct leading from the liver into the gallbladder (bile duct of Luschka). If this is found, it is identified, sealed, and clipped. Once the gallbladder is totally removed from the liver, it is held to one side and the liver bed is washed with saline to show up any bleeding points, which are sealed with heat or, sometimes, sutures.

❻ A moistened retrieval bag is inserted into the abdomen through one of the incisions and the gallbladder is tucked inside. The bag is then sealed and removed from the abdomen through either the belly button incision, or the cut below the ribs. Using a retrieval bag reduces the chance of spilling bile and stones during extraction. If the gallbladder has a large stone that cannot easily be removed through the small incision, it can be carefully crushed within the retrieval bag. After removal of the bag, a final inspection is made to check for bleeding or bile leaks. Then as much air as possible is deflated from the abdomen (to reduce post-operative pain) and the abdominal incisions are closed using sutures, skin tape, or staples.

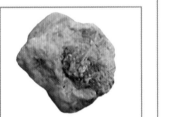

ABOVE A gallstone.

ABOVE RIGHT A gallbladder which has been removed surgically.

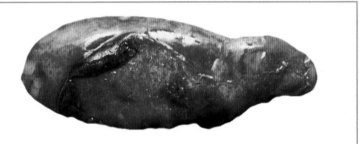

Some surgeons inject a long-acting local anesthetic into the sides of the wounds before closing to reduce post-operative discomfort. If there is concern about a possible bile leak, a drain may be left in place overnight to detect this as early as possible. This is not routinely needed, however.

Latest laparoscopic technique

In 2008, the first single-port cholecystectomy, using only a single incision in the umbilicus, was performed in the United States. A special device containing three ports was inserted into the umbilical incision through which all the necessary surgical instruments were inserted and manipulated. This has been hailed as signaling the next generation of minimally invasive surgery.

CHOLECYSTECTOMY
QUESTIONS & ANSWERS

What are the benefits?

Removal of the gallbladder prevents any further pain due to biliary colic or cholecystitis. It also reduces the potential risk of small gallstones triggering pancreatitis.

What are the risks?

As well as the general risks associated with surgery and general anesthesia *(see pages 10–11)*, complications include damage to the bile ducts and bile leakage which will need repair. An abscess may occasionally form under the liver.

Are there any alternatives?

Following the development of laparoscopic cholecystectomy, other treatments are now rarely used. Alternatives include extracorporeal (outside the body) shock-wave lithotripsy in which ultrasound is used to shatter a large stone so it can be passed naturally. Oral treatment with bile acids can dissolve cholesterol stones but it takes many months to work. In an older person who is not fit for surgery, gallstones or infected bile can be removed by opening the gallbladder using a small incision (percutaneous cholecystostomy) and draining the contents of the bladder through the abdominal wall.

Although these alternative options can remove current gallstones, the diseased gallbladder remains in place, and stones/infection can recur in the future.

What can I do to prepare?

People with gallstones are advised to follow a low fat, high fiber diet. This is because dietary fat acts as a trigger for contraction of the gallbladder, which may push a gallstone into the mouth of the bile duct to cause biliary colic. Healthy oils, such as olive oil and fish oil *(see page 35)*, may have a beneficial effect on bile. Drink plenty of fluids — especially water or herbal teas — to keep well hydrated; this helps to prevent sludging of bile which encourages gallstone formation. Keep alcohol intake to within recommended levels.

What if I don't have the operation?

Biliary colic due to gallstones or cholecystitis are likely to recur.

What happens during the recovery period?

The nasogastric tube is removed at the end of the operation before you wake up. You will usually breath oxygen via a mask for the first few hours. If a drain was inserted to check for bile leakage, this is usually removed the day after the operation if it remains clear. Most people are able to go home the day after a laparoscopic cholecystectomy, with suitable pain relief, for rest. After an open operation you may remain in

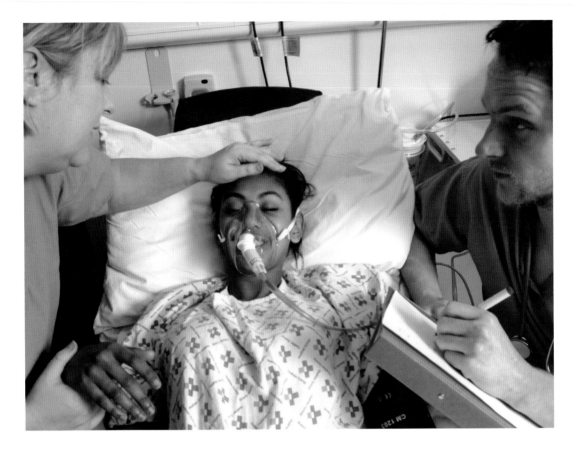

ABOVE A patient recovering from surgery with oxygen being supplied via a face mask.

hospital for four to five days. The wounds will have adhesive dressings which are usually kept on for a week. You can usually return to work seven to ten days following a laparoscopic cholecystectomy, and four weeks after an open operation if your job involves no heavy lifting. Air left in the abdomen can cause distension pain which is often referred to the shoulder.

As the gallbladder is merely a storage organ for bile made in the liver, it is a non-essential structure and most people do not miss it. After the gallbladder is removed, bile trickles down from the liver into the gut on a continual basis, rather than being stored en route and only squirted out after eating a fatty meal. This may cause no digestive problems, although some people develop bowel looseness or discomfort when eating certain foods as a result.

Diet

Olive oil is a rich source of monounsaturated fat which has a beneficial effect on blood cholesterol balance and bile composition. Use olive oil during cooking and in salad dressings. Omega-3 fish oils are also beneficial, so aim to eat oily fish (e.g. salmon, sardines, herrings) two or three times a week. Soluble fiber, such as pectins (e.g. found in apples, carrots) and gums (found in oat bran and beans), bind to cholesterol and bile salts in the gut to reduce their re-absorption and may help to reduce gallstone formation.

TONSILLECTOMY/ ADENOIDECTOMY

Tonsillectomy is the surgical removal of the tonsils, while adenoidectomy is the surgical removal of the adenoids. Although the two procedures are often performed together, either operation may be carried out alone.

WHAT ARE THE TONSILS AND ADENOIDS?

The tonsils and adenoids are areas of lymphoid tissue at the back of the throat (pharynx) with the adenoids situated, out of sight, above the tonsils. Healthy tonsils and adenoids produce white blood cells (lymphocytes) and antibodies that help to protect the nose and throat from infection. They are naturally large until around the age of five to seven years as young children are constantly exposed to bacteria and viruses to which they have not yet acquired immunity. After this age, the tonsils and adenoids slowly start to shrink.

Infection of the tonsils (tonsillitis) is usually due to common cold viruses or bacteria, such as beta-hemolytic streptococci. Symptoms vary, depending on severity, and can include feeling unwell with sore throat, unpleasant smelling breath, and painful swallowing with swelling and redness of the tonsils. Collections of pus may be seen within the crevices of the tonsillar surface *(see left)*.

If a tonsillar abscess (quinsy) develops, there is severe pain, swelling of the throat, and drooling due to difficulty swallowing. Speech may also be muffled (as if eating a hot potato). This is a surgical emergency as, if not drained, swelling may obstruct breathing.

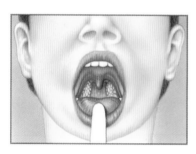

ABOVE Diagram of an opened child's mouth during an examination, showing enlarged, infected tonsils.

WHY ARE THEY REMOVED?

Tonsils are not usually removed unless absolutely necessary — and then rarely before the age of four as they are important for a child's immune defenses. Most cases of tonsillitis are self-limiting and improve with painkillers, fluid, and rest. If symptoms are severe or recurrent, so that a child misses a lot of school, tonsillectomy may be considered as diseased tonsils are less effective at fighting infection.

Good hygiene is essential

Tonsillitis is contagious and can be passed on through coughing, sneezing, and sharing food or utensils. Wash hands frequently, place a hand in front of the mouth before coughing (and wash afterward), avoid sharing cups and cutlery etc.

TONSILLECTOMY/ADENOIDECTOMY AT A GLANCE

- *Can it be done as an outpatient?* Yes, the majority are. Infants (under the age of three years), children with very large tonsils, obstructive sleep apnea, or suspected abscess are admitted to hospital.

- *Do I need a general anesthetic?* Usually, yes. Occasionally tonsillectomy is performed under a local anesthetic in adults.

- *What special tests are needed?* Throat swabs are taken to identify a bacterial infection (with beta-hemolytic streptococci) which is present in around 40% of children with tonsillitis. This is more likely if the temperature is over 100 °F (38 °C), common cold symptoms such as cough are absent, pus has collected on the tonsils, and neck glands are tender. It is not possible to definitely tell a bacterial from a viral tonsillitis on examination alone, however. Antibiotics (penicillin or erythromycin) are only prescribed if a streptococcal infection is confirmed, as viral infections are more common. If glandular fever (infectious mononucleosis) is suspected, this can be diagnosed with a blood test. Computed tomography (CT) scanning or magnetic resonance imaging (MRI) may be requested if an abscess is suspected. Adenoids may be evaluated with a side-view neck X-ray or with a viewing device (nasopharyngoscopy). You may have a blood test to check your blood clotting time as the main complication of tonsillectomy is heavy bleeding.

- *How long does the surgery take?* Around 20 to 30 minutes, or longer, depending on the extent of surgery.

- *What is the mortality rate?* Very low at around one in 15,000. One in 40,000 patients dies as a result of post-operative hemorrhage.

- *How long will I be in hospital?* Patients usually stay in hospital for an average of two to three days.

- *How expensive is it?* (\$)

- *How many are performed in the US each year?* Around 19,000 operations are performed annually as an inpatient. 740,000 tonsillectomies are performed as an outpatient, with or without adenoidectomy. 140,000 adenoidectomies are performed without tonsillectomy. Four out of five operations involve children under the age of 17 years.

The American Academy of Otolaryngology (Head and Neck Surgery) recommends that children who have three or more tonsil infections a year undergo a tonsillectomy.

The adenoids may be removed if persistent swelling causes problems with snoring, obstructive sleep apnea *(see below)*, or if they block off the drainage channel from the middle ear (Eustachian tube) or the sinuses to cause recurrent middle ear infections (otitis media) or sinusitis.

Obstructive sleep apnea

Obstructive sleep apnea can occur when enlarged tonsils or adenoids partially block the airway during sleep. This causes loud snoring and, when complete obstruction occurs, breathing stops. Failure to breathe causes carbon dioxide to build up in the blood, activating a survival mechanism in the brain that restarts the breathing process. As the airway is jerked open, a gasp occurs and you may briefly wake up. These episodes can lead to significant daytime problems if they last for more than ten seconds each time and occur more than ten times per night. In extreme cases, sleep apnea can happen as often as 100 to 1000 times per night, resulting in excessive daytime sleepiness.

TONSILLECTOMY/ADENOIDECTOMY
STEP-BY-STEP

TWO PHASE PROCEDURES

Although performed less often than previously, tonsillectomy remains one of the most common surgical procedures performed in childhood. The indications for surgery are controversial, and debate continues about which technique is best, and even whether tonsillectomy is better than conservative approaches such as antibiotics and pain relief. Several studies suggest that children who undergo tonsillectomy experience fewer throat infections, and fewer days off school over the following two years, than those managed conservatively with watchful waiting, however. In children with obstructive sleep apnea, surgery improves snoring and sleep disruption and one in four returns to normal sleep patterns.

Tonsillectomy and adenoidectomy are both two phase procedures that involve removal of tissues followed by control of bleeding (hemostasis). Some surgeons have started to use a technique called intracapsular tonsillectomy which leaves some tissue behind *(see page 41)* but most still use the traditional extracapsular approach which removes all tonsillar tissues.

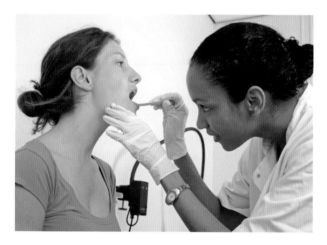

ABOVE A doctor examines the mouth of a patient suffering with painful tonsils.

❶ The operation is performed with the patient in Rose's position, in which you lie on your back, often with a roll under your shoulders, so your head falls backward over the end of the table. This helps to reduce the chance of inhaling blood into the lungs. The surgeon may sit with the patient's head in his or her lap to perform the operation. A mouth prop is inserted to keep the patient's mouth open *(see opposite left)*.

❷ The surgeon uses forceps to grasp the tonsil on one side *(see opposite right)*. Pulling on the forceps helps to lift the tonsil as it is carefully cut away. The surgeon dissects out and scrapes away tonsillar tissue, using his or her preferred instruments. Traditional approaches use blunt and sharp "cold steel" dissecting instruments, such as scissors, scalpel, a wire loop called a "snare," and/or a sharp spoon-shaped curette. Alternatives include using a hot blade

Dental inspection

The surgeon will inspect a child's teeth before starting to operate, and may remove any loose milk teeth in children who are shedding their first dentition. This prevents the danger of accidental dislodging and inhalation of a tooth during surgery.

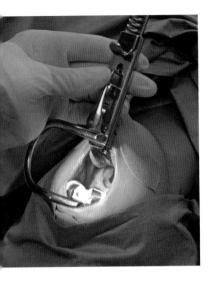

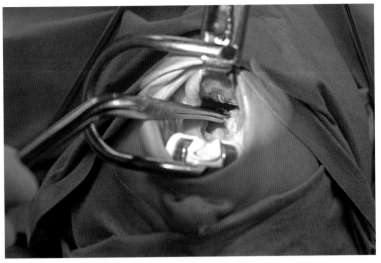

ABOVE A patient's mouth is clamped open during surgery.

ABOVE RIGHT The surgeon grasps the tonsil on one side with special forceps.

(electrocautery) which seals tissues as it cuts through. Electrocautery heats tissues to between 750 ° and 1110 °F (400 ° and 600 °C). This may burn deeper tissues to cause more post-operative discomfort. More advanced techniques include using a harmonic scalpel, in which ultrasound produces vibrations of 55,500 cycles per second within the blade. These rapid movements are invisible to the eye, but are transmitted to tissues to generate heat of between 120 ° and 210 °F (50 ° and 100 °C). This produces more precise cutting and coagulation with minimal risk of heat damage. A hot suction device can also be used to cut and seal tonsillar tissue (electrocautery) while simultaneously sucking away removed tissues. Another new technique, called thermal welding, uses both heat and pressure to seal and divide tissues; the tissue is grasped with forceps and a heating element is activated. This vaporizes tissues at temperatures of 570 ° to 750 °F (300 ° to 400 °C), and blood vessels are sealed by a combination of the clamping pressure of the forceps, plus the heat.

Using hot techniques reduces operative time and the risk of bleeding during surgery. However, some evidence suggests that traditional "cold steel" approaches result in less post-operative bleeding than the newer heat methods, and a faster return to a normal diet. Until these methods have been fully evaluated, many surgeons continue to use the older "tried and tested" techniques.

Variant Creutzfeldt Jacob Disease

Variant Creutzfeldt Jacob Disease (vCJD) is a rare, degenerative brain disorder that was first identified in 1996. It is a transmissible infection which, although not fully understood, has been linked with an infection marker found in the tonsils. There has been concern that vCJD may, theoretically, be transmitted through re-use of surgical instruments. In view of this theoretical risk, disposable, single-use instruments are often selected. There have been no reported cases of vCJD where tonsillectomy was the only possible cause, however.

STOPPING BLEEDING

❸ Bleeding, which can be copious, is stopped by applying pressure with a sponge, which may be dipped in epinephrine (to constrict blood vessels) or thrombin powder (which promotes clotting). Other methods include tying off bleeding vessels, or sealing them with heat (diathermy). Once the tonsil on one side is removed and bleeding is controlled, the surgeon repeats the procedure on the opposite tonsil.

RIGHT A surgeon uses electrocautery and forceps to dissect out the left tonsil.

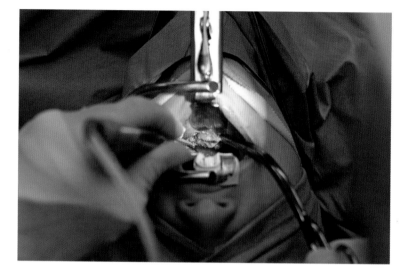

❹ If performing adenoidectomy, the surgeon uses a mirror to visualize the adenoids, which are hidden behind the nasal cavity *(see below)*. Adenoidectomy is performed using specialized steel instruments with long handles. An adenoid curette has a sharp cutting edge, an adenoid punch has a chamber that is placed over the adenoid tissue. When closed, a blade cuts off the tissue which falls into the chamber for removal. Adenoid forceps are used to remove residual tissue. A hot suction device can also be used to cut and seal adenoid tissue

RIGHT A surgeon uses a mirror coated with an anti-mist agent to view the adenoids as they are treated with a hot suction device (blue) to shrink them.

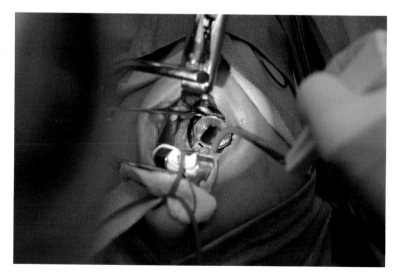

(electrocautery) while simultaneously sucking away removed tissues *(see below)*. An alternative approach is to remove the adenoids by operating through the nasal cavity with a suction microdebrider.

❺ Bleeding of the adenoid bed is controlled by nasal packing and heat sealing (electrocautery). If bleeding is persistent, or recurs, a post-nasal pack may be left in place for four to 24 hours after surgery.

❻ If significant bleeding occurred during surgery, the stomach may be emptied with a nasogastric tube to reduce the possibility of post-operative nausea and vomiting.

BELOW A surgeon finishes treating the adenoids with a hot suction device (blue). Blood loss can be extensive during this operation, and must be carefully controlled.

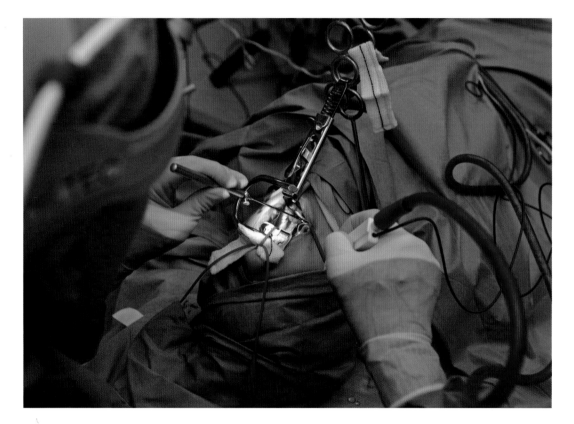

Intracapsular tonsillectomy

Intracapsular tonsillectomy does not remove the whole tonsil but 90% to 95% of the tissue, leaving the thin outer layer (capsule) of the tonsil in place so the underlying throat muscles are not exposed. This is achieved using an electrically powered endoscopic instrument called a microdebrider, which rotates to shave tonsil tissue away. The shavings are removed using a continuous suction device. The remaining tonsillar capsule acts as a biological dressing to reduce inflammation and infection. Intracapsular tonsillectomy is less likely to cause bleeding after surgery, and discomfort is also reduced. In some cases the remaining tonsillar tissue regrows so that further surgery is needed for persistent tonsillitis in the future, but this appears to occur in less than one in 100 cases.

TONSILLECTOMY/ADENOIDECTOMY
QUESTIONS & ANSWERS

What are the benefits?

Removal of enlarged tonsils and/or adenoids can improve or solve related problems, such as recurrent throat infections, middle ear infections (otitis media), glue ear, nasal voice, snoring, or sleep apnea.

What are the risks?

As well as the general risks associated with surgery and general anesthesia *(see pages 10–11)*, there is a risk of heavy bleeding as the tonsils are highly vascular. Significant bleeding within 24 hours (primary hemorrhage) occurs in around one in 100 patients. The risk of bleeding within one day and ten days after surgery (secondary hemorrhage) is between one and seven per 100 (1%–7%). In around one in 250 patients, bleeding is severe enough to warrant a return to theater. One in 40,000 patients undergoing tonsillectomy dies as a result of bleeding. After adenoidectomy, there may be temporary changes in voice after surgery due to incomplete closure of the soft palate. Rarely, this is persistent.

Are there any alternatives?

Drinking iced drinks or eating ice cream can help to relieve symptoms of tonsillitis, acetaminophen will ease pain, and antibiotics are indicated if the infection is due to a bacterial rather than a viral infection. A humidifier or steam inhalations may help to ease breathing. For adults, other procedures may be available that use lasers, radiofrequency ablation, or a form of plasma energy (coblation) to heat tonsil tissues to 104 °–158 °F (40–70 °C), causing them to shrink. These new methods are still being evaluated to determine their effectiveness, however. Topical nasal steroid spray and saline spray may help to reduce nasal obstruction due to enlarged adenoids.

What can I do to prepare?

Try to be as fit as possible. If you smoke, do your utmost to stop as this increases the chance of infection and reduces healing.

What if I don't have the operation?

Tonsillitis and/or swelling of the adenoids may recur or persist. Swollen adenoids may cause a worsening nasal voice, snoring, and sleep apnea. The tonsil and adenoid tissues will eventually shrink as you get older, however. Many physicians encourage a "watchful waiting" approach to try to avoid surgery.

What happens during the recovery period?

You are lain on your side after the operation to prevent inhalation of blood into the lungs. The throat feels very sore after surgery, and regular painkillers are needed. You may develop a stiff or cricked neck (torticollis) due to spasm of neck muscles. This resolves with warm compresses, anti-inflammatory drugs, and the temporary use of a soft neck brace.

For the first 24 hours, you will need a light diet of fluids and soft, pureed food as swallowing is painful. Ice cream is a popular choice as the cold helps to soothe the area. It is important to observe children closely as they may become dehydrated or lose weight through not eating or drinking enough due to pain.

Following tonsillectomy, pain usually reduces during the first three to five days, then increases for one or two days before resolving. A white scab forms over the tonsil bed, usually five to ten days after surgery, as part of the healing process. You may experience a temporary nasal voice.

Avoid heavy lifting for ten days.

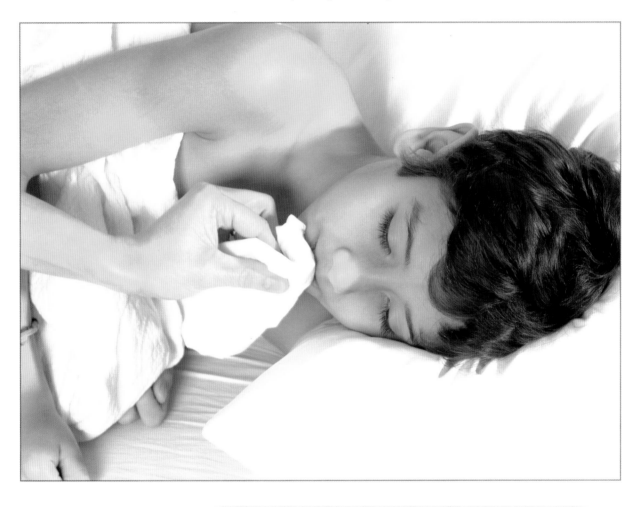

ABOVE A child recovers at home after a tonsillectomy.

Important note

Contact your doctor straight away if you experience bleeding, earache, or high fever after going home.

CARPAL TUNNEL RELEASE

Carpal tunnel release is the surgical loosening of a bony tunnel in the wrist to free a trapped nerve. The carpal tunnel is a narrow space found between bones in the wrist that are covered by a strong band of tissue, the transverse carpal ligament. The median nerve passes through this space, together with nine flexor tendons that bend the fingers and thumb. Because of this overcrowding in an anatomically narrow area, the median nerve can become pinched which causes painful tingling and sensations that resemble an electric shock. Known as median neuropathy, or carpal tunnel syndrome (CTS), symptoms classically involve the thumb, index, and middle fingers plus the inner side of the ring finger, as these areas are supplied by the median nerve. In severe cases, numbness, weakness, and muscle wasting may also occur.

WHO GETS CARPAL TUNNEL SYNDROME?

CTS most commonly affects women, as the female carpal tunnel is anatomically smaller than that of males. Heredity is another important factor, as having a tight carpal tunnel can run in some families. It is also associated with obesity, in which fatty tissue can cause further restriction, and with a number of other conditions associated with weight gain or tissue swelling *(see below)*. Often, however, no obvious underlying risk factors are identified.

Although there is no consensus on whether specific work activities can cause CTS, some people believe their symptoms are brought on by repetitive finger movements, such as those involved in typing or playing a musical instrument. During these movements, tendons in the wrist slide to-and-fro inside their sheaths and, if the wrist is held in an awkward position (cocked up, down, or to one side)

CTS is associated with:
- Obesity.
- Pregnancy.
- Menopause.
- Underactive thyroid gland (hypothyroidism).
- Type 2 diabetes.
- Arthritis, especially rheumatoid arthritis.
- Previous wrist fracture.
- Kidney failure.
- Acromegaly (in which a pituitary gland tumor secretes growth hormone).
- Taking certain drugs, including oral contraceptives.

CARPAL TUNNEL RELEASE AT A GLANCE

- **Can it be done as an outpatient?** Yes. Almost all carpal tunnel releases are performed in an outpatient setting.

- **Do I need a general anesthetic?** Many people are able to have the operation under local anesthesia *(see page 46)* and light sedation. General anesthesia is also an option.

- **What special tests are needed?** X-rays of the wrist may be indicated if you have limited wrist movements or previous fracture. Nerve conduction studies can confirm the diagnosis by demonstrating a slower than normal speed of conduction within the median nerve. Ultrasound or magnetic resonance imaging (MRI) is sometimes used to evaluate the soft tissues in the carpal tunnel.

- **How long does the surgery take?** Usually between 15 to 20 minutes. More complicated cases can take up to an hour or more.

- **What is the mortality rate?** Less than 0.25% (one in 400).

- **How long will I be in hospital?** Surgery is usually performed within one day on an outpatient basis.

- **How expensive is it?** 💲

- **How many are performed in the US each year?** Around 580,000 operations are performed in the US each year, with three times more women requiring surgery than males.

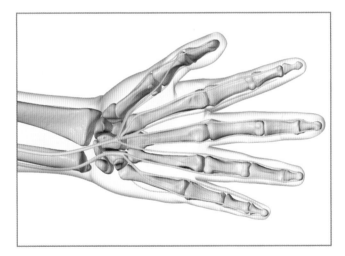

this may lead to inflammation and swelling of tissues around the sheaths (peritendonitis and tenosynovitis) to put pressure on the median nerve. Another explanation is that repetitive movements affect the muscles and nerve endings in the hand and forearm to cause pain of a biomechanical nature rather than through a true carpal tunnel syndrome. This is a controversial area, as it can affect entitlement to time off work and financial compensation.

LEFT Nerves supplying the hand pass over the carpal bones in the wrist.

Testing for carpal tunnel syndrome

Doctors may perform a few clinical tests if they suspect CTS.
- Phalen's maneuver involves gently flexing the wrists by placing the hands back to back and holding them there for 60 seconds, to see if this brings on symptoms.
- Eliciting Tinel's sign involves tapping lightly over the median nerve at the crease in the wrist to see if this causes tingling or pins and needles.
- Durkan's test involves applying firm pressure over the carpal tunnel for 30 seconds to see if this brings on symptoms.
- Asking you to try to straighten your thumb against resistance checks for weakness of the median nerve.
- Touching your fingertips with a pin checks whether or not you can distinguish between one and two pin points, held close together, with your eyes closed.

CARPAL TUNNEL RELEASE
STEP-BY-STEP

OPEN HAND SURGERY

Open carpal tunnel release is the most commonly performed operation for CTS, although an endoscopic surgical technique is available *(see page 49)*. Open surgery provides better visualization of the median nerve and is preferred by many hand surgeons because of the reduced risk of median nerve damage. It also allows the surgeon to divide the outermost layer of tissue surrounding the nerve (epineurium) if necessary to free a tightly trapped nerve in a procedure called epineurolysis. It also allows him or her to remove any excess tissue surrounding the flexor tendons in a procedure called flexor tenosynovectomy; this is needed if symptoms are linked with swelling or a build up of scar tissue.

As carpal tunnel release is usually carried out under local anesthetic, you will remain awake throughout the short operation. Light sedation may be offered which means you are likely to remember very little of the procedure afterward.

BELOW A surgeon and assistant prepare to start a carpal tunnel release operation on an anesthetized patient.

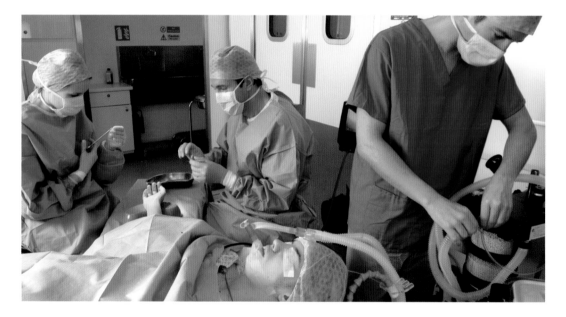

Local anesthesia for carpal tunnel release

The hand and wrist can be numbed in several ways. Local anesthetic can be injected into the tissues at the site of surgery; local anesthetic can be injected into veins in the lower arm (intravenous regional anesthesia), or most of the arm can be numbed by injecting local anesthetic around nerves in the armpit or elbow (peripheral nerve block). When a tourniquet is applied to maintain a bloodless operative field, this helps to prolong pain relief by slowing the amount of local anesthetic agent flushed away. Although local injection of anesthetic agent into the tissues is the easiest option, it does not provide enough pain relief if epineurolysis or flexor tenosynovectomy are needed.

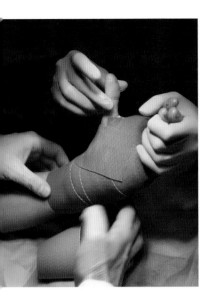

You will be asked to sit in a chair, or lie on an operating table with your arm resting out to the side. The surgeon will use a pen to mark out the important anatomical landmarks on your skin. Local anesthesia is used to numb the wrist and palm. A tight tourniquet is applied to your arm and, in some cases, is slowly wrapped up from your fingers to remove most of the blood from your lower arm (limb exsanguination) *(see left)*. This allows the surgeon to operate in a bloodless field, which is essential for a clear view to reduce the risk of median nerve injury. It also helps to keep the local anesthetic agent in the area, and is essential if you are having intravenous regional anesthesia *(see page 46)*.

ABOVE Theater assistants apply a bandage to squeeze blood out of the patient's hand before surgery is initiated.

❶ The surgeon makes a straight incision over the palm of your hand, in line with your ring finger. The cut extends down to just above the first wrist crease, and is sometimes longer if greater exposure is needed. The incision is usually 1.5 in to 3 in (4 cm to 8 cm) long.

❷ The fat beneath the skin is pulled to either side with retractors to expose the underlying sheet-like tissue, called the superficial palmar fascia. This is cut through in line with the skin incision, and also retracted to either side, to expose the underlying transverse carpal ligament.

BELOW A carpal tunnel release operation in progress.

❸ The surgeon passes a blunt, curved clamp under the ligament to protect the nerve and flexor tendons beneath. Using the clamp as a guide, the surgeon carefully cuts the transverse carpal ligament along its length, under direct vision.

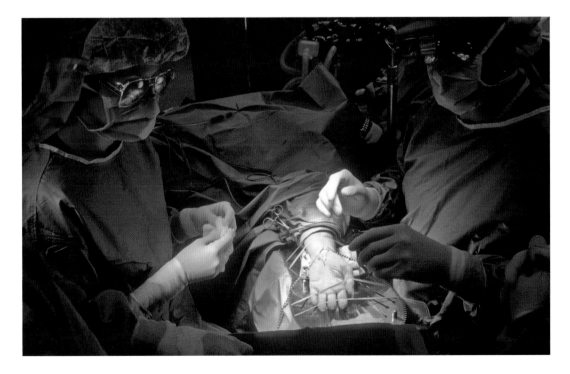

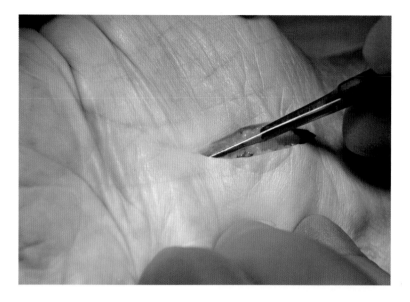

❹ A blunt instrument is then used to loosen a sheet-like tissue at the wrist, the deep fascia of the forearm, which is connected to the transverse carpal ligament. This tissue is also cut longitudinally, for 0.8 in to 1.2 in (2 cm to 3 cm), up toward the forearm *(see below)*. If the surgeon cannot see this tissue properly, he or she may need to extend the palm incision down over the wrist, at an angle, to make a J-shaped cut.

❺ Once the surgeon is satisfied that the carpal tunnel is sufficiently freed up, the tourniquet is released so that blood can flow back into the area. Any bleeding points are sealed shut with heat (electrocautery).

❻ The skin incision is closed with sutures and a sterile dressing applied over the wound.

RIGHT The surgeon cuts the transverse carpal ligament to ease pressure within the carpal tunnel.

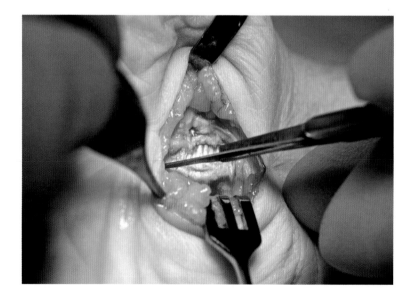

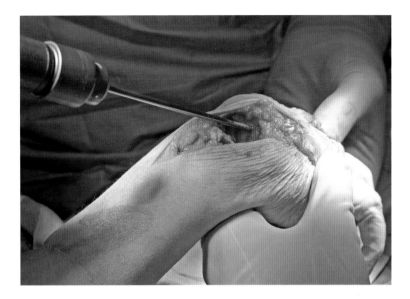

Endoscopic carpal tunnel release

Minimally invasive surgery aims to cut the transverse carpal ligament from within the carpal tunnel, leaving the overlying structures intact. This can be carried out through either one, or two, small incisions. In both techniques, the first incision is 0.6 in (1.5 cm) wide, and is made at the base of the forearm, just in front of the first wrist crease. The underlying loose tissue is carefully dissected and spread apart to preserve any tiny nerves. A flap, rather like a trap-door, is cut into the underlying deep fascia of the forearm, to expose the carpal tunnel. Blunt probes are then inserted to gently open up a passage through the tunnel.

Single incision technique: A combined viewing and cutting device is inserted and advanced down toward the palm to the correct position. The underside of the transverse carpal ligament is easily identified as it is made up of striped bands of collagen. The blade is raised and the device carefully withdrawn to cut through the ligament. Two or three passes are needed to complete the procedure. The device is then reinserted to check that the ligament is fully divided. Finally, the device is inserted in the other direction, up toward the forearm, and manipulated to cut the lower part of the deep fascia of the forearm, which is connected to the transverse carpal ligament.

Two incision technique: If two small incisions are used, the second is made parallel to the first, in the lower palm. A clear, plastic sheath is then passed into the wrist incision, through the carpal tunnel, to the palm incision, through which the viewing device (endoscope) is inserted. The transverse carpal ligament is then cut with a special, reverse cutting knife placed in the other end of the sheath, which the surgeon can see through the endoscope. The endoscope and knife are then withdrawn. The surgeon then re-inserts them in the opposite direction, so the endoscope enters the sheath from the palm incision, and the knife through the wrist incision. The deep fascia of the forearm is then cut.

Once the surgeon is satisfied that the carpal tunnel is sufficiently freed, the tourniquet is released so that blood can flow back into the area. Any bleeding points are sealed and the skin incision(s) closed with sutures. If, at any time, the surgeon is unable to see properly what he or she is cutting, endoscopy is abandoned and the operation converted to an open carpal tunnel release. Endoscopic carpal tunnel release surgery typically takes 30 to 45 minutes to complete.

CARPAL TUNNEL RELEASE
QUESTIONS & ANSWERS

What are the benefits?

Nine out of ten people experience greatly improved symptoms following surgery, though recovery is gradual, and it can take several months or even a year to regain full grip strength.

What are the risks?

As well as the general risks associated with surgery *(see pages 10–11)*, there is a small risk of surgical damage to the median nerve and tendons running within the carpal tunnel, or of cutting a blood vessel such as the ulnar artery. Recurrent scar formation is the most common complication. Incomplete release of the transverse carpal ligament and deep fascia of the forearm can occur, and is most likely with endoscopic procedures. Carpal tunnel syndrome can recur in between 7% and 20% of people and revision surgery is usually less successful than the original operation.

Are there any alternatives?

Painkillers and anti-inflammatory drugs can reduce discomfort. Pressure may be reduced by wearing wrist splints at night. Those which hold the wrist at a neutral angle may be more effective at relieving pain than those that hold the wrist in an upward, bent position. Steroid injections may be suggested. Some people with CTS have a low vitamin B6 level and, although supplements are not effective in everyone, some people improve with supplements. An estimated one third of people do not respond to conservative approaches.

What can I do to prepare?

Exercises can help to free up the median nerve, which travels through a distance of 0.8 in (2 cm) between wrist flexion and distension. Try curling your fingers up into a fist and bending your wrist toward your palm, then straighten your fingers and stretch your wrist back the other way. Repeat this ten times, whenever you feel the need. If you smoke, do your utmost to stop to reduce the risk of infection (smoking lowers natural immunity) and to hasten recovery.

Balloon carpal tunnel-plasty

A newly developed surgical procedure aims to relieve symptoms of CTS without cutting the transverse carpal ligament. A small incision is made in the base of the palm and a catheter containing a small balloon is inserted under the ligament. The balloon is inflated with saline to stretch the ligament and ease pressure within the carpal tunnel. In one study, patients returned to work within two weeks.

What if I don't have the operation?

Symptoms may resolve with conservative approaches, including losing any excess weight. Symptoms may worsen, however, and pain may wake you at night. Progressive muscle weakness and wasting may develop as a result of persistent median nerve compression. This may prevent you from grasping objects.

What happens during the recovery period?

You will usually wear a post-operative splint for four to ten days until the sutures are removed. You may then wear a wrist splint or glove until the pain subsides. You may be advised to elevate your hand and perform exercises that move your fingers to minimize swelling and stiffness. Recovery time depends on the severity of symptoms and the degree of compression to which the median nerve was subjected. Pain in the palm of the hand is common for several months. The average time to return to work is five weeks. People whose work involves bending and twisting of the hands and wrists tend to return to work later than those whose work does not involve particular hand movements. You should avoid heavy lifting and repetitive movements for six to eight weeks.

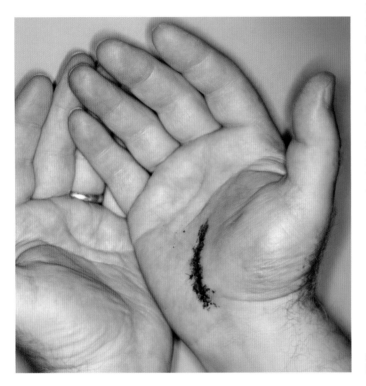

LEFT The stitched wound on a man's hand heals after carpal tunnel surgery.

Lifestyle modifications

An ergonomic assessment of work conditions is essential as altering posture, chair, and table heights, computer placement, and the correct use of a keyboard can improve symptoms.

- Take regular breaks from tasks requiring repetitive movements — try not to sit still for more than 20 minutes.
- Stretch arms back, upward, and forward while sitting, and circle elbows to your sides.
- When using a keyboard, your shoulders should be relaxed, your upper arm vertical, forearm horizontal, and your wrist in a neutral, balanced position — not cocked upward.
- Ergonomically designed keyboards with specially shaped key pads and integral wrist rests are available.
- Most people use excessive grip for tasks. Learn to relax your grip (e.g. when holding a phone) and use less force (for example, when typing).
- Avoid bending your wrist excessively up or down — use a wrist rest when typing.
- Keep your hands warm.

Inguinal Hernia Repair

A hernia repair operation is known as a herniorrhaphy. A hernia occurs when an internal part of the body pushes through a weakness in the tissues that normally contain it. This forms an external bulge which is sometimes referred to as a rupture. In the case of an inguinal hernia, a part of the intestines pushes through a weakness between the abdomen and the top of the leg in the region of the inguinal canal. This area is weaker in men than in women, as the spermatic cord passes through and dilates the inguinal canal on each side, on its way into the scrotum. Inguinal hernias are, therefore, more common in men than in women.

Direct and indirect inguinal hernias

There are two main types: indirect inguinal hernias pass down through the inguinal canal, and may extend into the scrotum (in males) or vulva (in females). Direct inguinal hernias push directly through a weakness in the lower abdominal wall, to one side of the inguinal canal, and hardly ever go down into the scrotum. A direct and indirect inguinal hernia may occur at the same time, and are known as pantaloon hernias because of the way they balloon and overlap around large blood vessels present in the area.

What causes an inguinal hernia?

A hernia is often triggered when an increase in abdominal pressure causes the inguinal canal weakness to give way. This may be due to persistent coughing, lifting heavy objects, or straining with constipation. Being overweight also increases the risk of a hernia as it places greater strain on any area of potential weakness and may also cause it to distend. Inguinal hernias can occur at any age, but are most likely to form in the first few months of life, in the late teens/early twenties, and between the ages of 40 and 60.

What are the symptoms?

If the external hernia develops suddenly, you may notice a sensation of something giving way, plus some discomfort or pain that usually improves. Otherwise, you may just notice the appearance of an unusual bulge or lump in the groin. The lump will feel soft and usually bulges when you cough.

If the hernia is reducible, the bulge can be gently pushed back into place and will disappear when you lie down. If the hernia cannot be

INGUINAL HERNIA REPAIR AT A GLANCE

• *Can it be done as an outpatient?* Yes, if it is a small, reducible, inguinal hernia. Large hernias, and those that are irreducible or showing signs of strangulation, require admission to hospital.

• *Do I need a general anesthetic?* Simple herniorrhaphy can be performed under local anesthesia and sedation. More complex hernias, and laparoscopic hernia repairs, are performed under general anesthesia or epidural *(see page 57)*.

• *What special tests are needed?* The hernia is examined while you are standing and lying down, and while you cough. An expansile cough impulse, which causes a groin lump to become larger and more tense, confirms it is a hernia rather than, for example, a fibrous lump or cyst. The surgeon will try to push the lump back into place, using slow constant pressure. Ice or cold compresses may be applied for several minutes to reduce swelling and allow easier reduction. The surgeon may listen to the hernia with a stethoscope to detect any bowel sounds. These

tests assess whether the hernia is reducible, trapped (incarcerated), or if it contains bowel. Ultrasound can also determine hernia contents.

• *How long does the surgery take?* A simple, open, tension-free repair takes 30 to 40 minutes. More complicated repairs of a large or irreducible hernia may take one hour or more.

• *What is the mortality rate?* Less than one in 100 (0.9%).

• *How long will I be in hospital?* Most hernias are repaired as a day case. For more complicated hernias, average hospital stay is five to six days.

• *How expensive is it?* $

• *How many are performed in the US each year?* Around 35,000 operations are performed as an inpatient each year. A further 528,000 inguinal hernia operations are performed as an outpatient. Four out of five operations are on males.

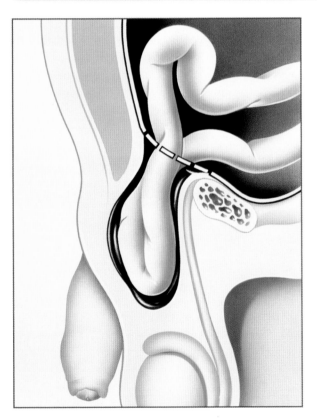

reduced — either because it is too large, or because the hole through which it has passed is too narrow — it may become trapped and painful. If the blood supply to the trapped intestine becomes cut off — a condition known as a strangulated hernia — severe pain occurs and you may also develop signs of intestinal obstruction, such as vomiting, abdominal pain, distension, or constipation. This is a surgical emergency that needs urgent treatment to free the trapped bowel. If you have an inguinal hernia and the lump becomes painful, contact your doctor straight away, as it may be trapped and in danger of losing its blood supply.

LEFT An illustration showing a loop of small intestine within an indirect inguinal hernia.

INGUINAL HERNIA REPAIR
STEP-BY-STEP

TENSION-FREE HERNIA REPAIR

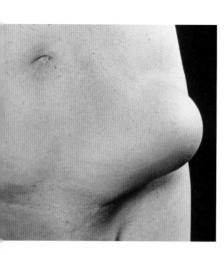

ABOVE **A man with an indirect inguinal hernia.**

Inguinal hernias vary in size from a bulge of 0.4 in (1 cm) in diameter, to a large mass that extends down as far as the knees. The bulge of an inguinal hernia contains a sac (made of peritoneal membrane that lines the abdominal cavity) plus one or more loops of small intestine, or a piece of fatty membrane (omentum) that is attached to the outside of the small intestines. A herniorrhaphy involves replacing the hernia contents in their correct anatomical position, then repairing the weakness through which they protruded so the hernia does not recur.

As the hernia may not be obvious once you are lying down, the surgeon usually marks the site of the hernia with a pen before the operation. Bilateral hernias can be repaired at the same time, or as two separate procedures.

Traditional hernia repairs merely pushed the intestines back into place then stitched together the two sides of the gap through which the hernia formed *(see opposite)*. These stitches were placed under tension, like a darn, to hold the wound together. This approach often caused persistent discomfort and an estimated 20% chance of the hernia recurring. Nowadays, most inguinal hernias are repaired using an open, tension-free reinforcement in which a piece of sterile, non-absorbable, polypropylene mesh is placed over the inguinal canal to cover the hernia opening. This prosthesis encourages strong, fibrous tissue to grow around and through the mesh. This quickly develops into a strong, tension-free reinforcement which, because it is inside the abdominal wall, means the hernia is less likely to recur.

The standard procedure for repairing an inguinal hernia involves an open, anterior approach. Laparoscopic repair *(see page 57)* is becoming more popular for young, otherwise fit, adults, as it allows a more rapid recovery and return to work.

RIGHT **Surgeons dissect out a hernia during repair in a Day Surgery Unit.**

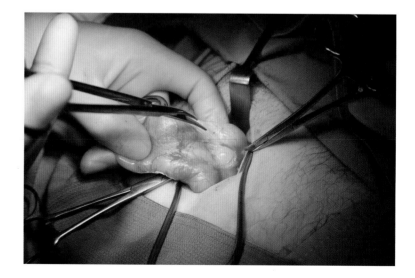

If performed under local anesthesia, the surgeon injects local anesthetic with epinephrine (which constricts blood vessels to reduce bleeding) along the line of the proposed incision. A small needle is used to numb the skin, then a larger needle is used to inject local anesthetic more deeply to block the nerves supplying the inguinal canal region. Half the anesthetic is reserved to inject around the neck of the peritoneal sac containing the hernia, and any other sensitive areas. Sedation is often used, too, so you remember little of the procedure afterward.

❶ An incision is made within a skin crease, usually starting a finger's breadth above the pubic bone. The incision is around 2.4 in (6 cm) long and extends two thirds of the way up to the hip bone. The surgeon cuts through the underlying tissue, sealing and cutting any large veins, while taking care not to cut into any intestines within the hernia.

❷ The surgeon identifies the exit leading from the inguinal canal (the external inguinal ring) and splits the fibrous tissue over the inguinal canal down as far as this point, to open the ring. Care is taken not to damage the nerve that runs in this area, which might cause numbness or pain after the operation.

❸ In male patients, the surgeon mobilizes the spermatic cord that passes through the inguinal canal, and carefully cuts down through the tissue covering it to expose the hernia. An indirect hernia is situated deeper within these tissues than a direct hernia, so the spermatic cord is thicker than its normal pencil-sized width. Even if an obvious direct hernia is present, the surgeon will cut into the tissues surrounding the spermatic cord to check for a simultaneous indirect hernia. An unsuspected additional hernia is found in 10% of operations. The surgeon also examines the abdominal wall to check for weaknesses that may lead to further hernias in the future.

RIGHT A hernia repair involving blue nylon sutures.

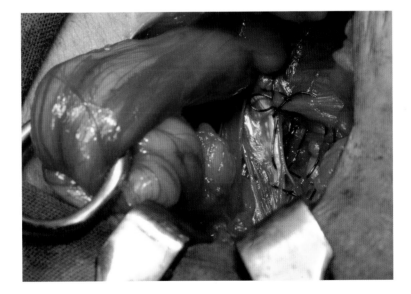

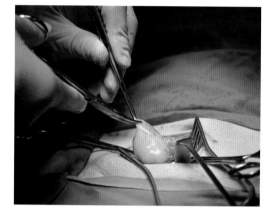

❹ The sac of the hernia is carefully peeled away from surrounding tissues and freed back to the level of the peritoneum that lines the abdominal cavity *(see left)*. The sac is then carefully opened and any contents gently returned to the peritoneal cavity if they haven't already slithered back on their own. The neck of the sac is then sewn closed and the stump pushed back into the abdomen. In an infant, this cutting of the hernia sac (herniotomy) may be all that is required, in which case the surgeon now closes the incision. Usually, however, the abdominal wall is also reinforced.

❺ A piece of polypropylene mesh (approximately 4.3 in/ 11 cm long by 2.4 in/6 cm wide) is placed over the entire inguinal canal region. In males, a small slit is cut in the mesh to accommodate the spermatic cord. The mesh is then stitched to hold it firmly in place *(see below)*.

ABOVE Surgeons removing fatty tissue from around a hernia sac.

❻ The tissue over the mesh is closed with absorbable stitches to re-form the external inguinal ring. The overlying skin is then closed with sutures, clips, staples, or adhesive strips.

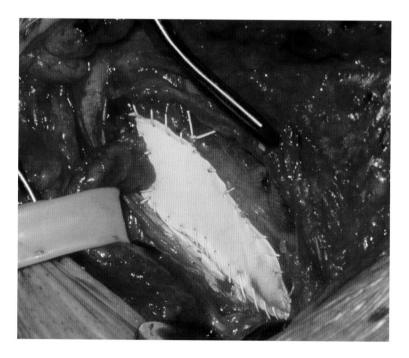

RIGHT A tension-free hernia repair involving a mesh.

Dome mesh

Instead of using a sheet of polypropylene mesh, some surgeons use a pre-formed dome of mesh, pushing it up the inguinal canal to cover the internal inguinal ring or other area of weakness.

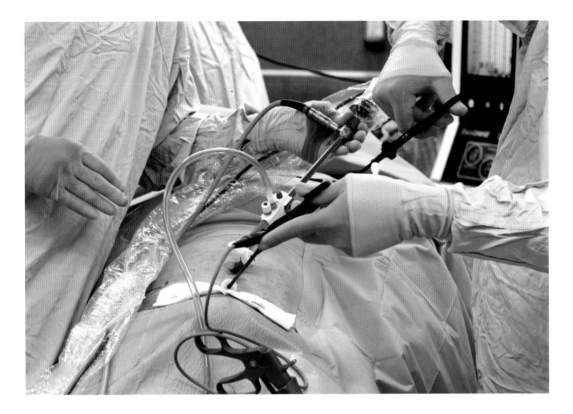

ABOVE Surgeons performing laparoscopic surgery (keyhole surgery) to repair an inguinal hernia.

Laparoscopic hernia repair

Minimally invasive, laparoscopic hernia repair is especially suitable for obese people who have a lot of stretched, fatty abdominal tissues, and for repairing bilateral and recurrent inguinal hernias. This may be performed by entering the abdominal cavity through the peritoneal membrane (trans-abdominal preperitoneal hernia repair, also known as TAPP) or by staying outside the peritoneum (totally extraperitoneal hernia repair, or TEP).

Tapp repair: During a TAPP repair, an incision is made above the umbilicus (belly button) through which carbon dioxide is pumped into the abdominal cavity, followed by insertion of the laparoscope (viewing device). Two further small incisions are made to insert the operating instruments — these sites vary depending on surgeon preference. The hernia is reduced by careful pulling. An incision is then made in the peritoneal membrane and a piece of mesh inserted

between the peritoneum and abdominal wall to cover the whole extent of the inguinal canal.

TEP repair: During a TEP repair, an incision is made in the abdominal wall below the umbilicus, and a balloon inflated between the peritoneal membrane and abdominal wall to create a space. The balloon is then removed, and the space enlarged by pumping in carbon dioxide gas. Two further, small incisions are made to insert the operating instruments — one above the pubic bone, and one on the side opposite the hernia (or opposite the largest hernia if they are bilateral). After reducing the hernia, a large sheet of mesh is inserted into the extraperitoneal space and stapled into place to cover the inguinal canal area. The mesh is held in place as the space is then slowly deflated.

With both procedures, the small skin incisions are closed with sutures and adhesive strips.

INGUINAL HERNIA REPAIR
QUESTIONS & ANSWERS

What are the benefits?

Repairing an inguinal hernia can reduce discomfort and remove an unsightly bulge. It also takes away the risk of a hernia becoming strangulated in the future.

What are the risks?

As well as the general risks associated with surgery and general anesthesia *(see pages 10–11)*, there is a risk of extensive bruising if blood vessels are damaged. There is a risk of producing a blood-filled lump (hematoma), especially in the case of a large hernia that extends down into the scrotum. Rarely, the spermatic cord may be damaged or constricted, leading to poor blood supply to the testicle (ischemic orchitis) which, if not recognized and corrected, may affect fertility. If nerves in the area are damaged, this may result in persistent groin pain or numbness. Most men experience no long term problems, however. The hernia may recur, but in a study involving over 3000 open, tension-free reinforcements, only eight recurrences occurred within an 18 month to five year follow up.

Are there any alternatives?

The traditional treatment for an inguinal hernia involves wearing a supportive truss. The hernia may be left as part of an approach called "watchful waiting" *(see below)*.

What can I do to prepare?

Try to ensure that you are as fit as possible, by exercising regularly and trying to lose any excess weight. If you smoke, do your utmost to stop, as smoking increases the risk of blood clots, infection, and impairs the healing process.

What if I don't have the operation?

Adult hernias will not heal by themselves and, if left untreated, may gradually become larger when they can cause discomfort and dragging sensations. A hernia is also at risk of becoming trapped and strangulated. However, men with a small inguinal hernia that is easily reducible, and which causes minimal symptoms, do not appear to experience significantly more pain, discomfort, or interference with everyday life if managed with "watchful waiting" than if the hernia is repaired. Your surgeon may therefore agree that you can delay surgical repair until symptoms warrant it.

What happens during the recovery period?

There is no stitching directly into the muscle and, because there is no tension, post-operative discomfort is usually minimal. A non-steroidal anti-inflammatory drug (NSAID) (e.g. diclofenac) inserted as a rectal suppository at the end of the operation (with your consent) is highly effective as pain relief if you do not have asthma or peptic ulcers, which are contraindications.

When a small hernia is repaired under local anesthetic, the procedure may take as little as 20 minutes, and patients can walk away afterward without needing to rest in bed. Oral NSAIDs may be taken for pain relief for a few days if needed, but one in five do not need any painkillers after surgery. Many patients are able to go for a walk or even a gentle jog the day after the operation as they start getting back into their normal routine.

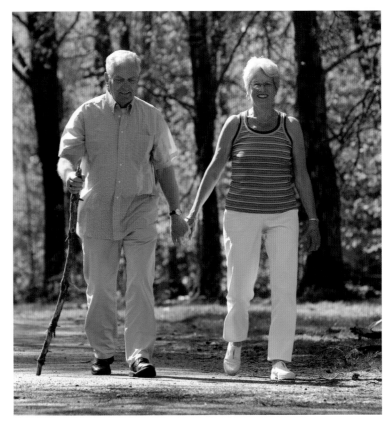

RIGHT Gentle exercise, such as walking, is possible soon after a tension-free hernia repair.

Returning to normal

- Avoid lifting heavy objects for at least one month.
- You can drive as soon as you can make an emergency stop without discomfort — usually after ten days.
- You can restart sexual activity as soon as the wound is comfortable — usually within a week.
- Those with sedentary jobs can return to work within a day or two following a tension-free repair, and within two weeks following a traditional stitch repair.
- Average time taken to return to work for manual workers is nine days.

KNEE REPLACEMENT (ARTHROPLASTY)

Knee replacement is performed when a knee joint is damaged by osteoarthritis. The knee joint occurs between the upper end of the tibia (shin bone), the lower end of the femur (thigh bone), and the back of the kneecap (patella). The bony surfaces within the joint are normally protected by slippery cartilage, and oiled by synovial fluid which cushions knee movements. The ends of the tibia and femur are further protected by two, crescent-shaped disks of cartilage, the medial and lateral menisci, which act like washers to reduce friction when the bones move together.

WHAT IS OSTEOARTHRITIS?

Osteoarthritis (OA) develops when the quality of cartilage and synovial fluid deteriorate. Although traditionally thought of as a wear-and-tear disease, researchers now believe that OA results from the active repair of damaged joints, when more cartilage is broken down than normal, but less new cartilage is made to replace it, so repair is incomplete. The cartilage becomes weaker, stiffer, and less able to withstand compressive forces. As a result, the articular cartilage protecting the bone ends becomes pitted, cracked, and starts to flake away to expose the underlying bone. When articular cartilage is lost, synovial fluid leaks into the underlying bone causing mild inflammation, bone thickening, and the formation of small cysts and bony outgrowths known as osteophytes. More and more cartilage is lost and, in severe cases, very little cartilage may remain.

WHO IS AFFECTED?

Osteoarthritis becomes more common with increasing age. This is because your cartilage becomes thinner and increasingly stiff and non-flexible as you get older, and because the progressive joint damage that

---

Symptoms of knee osteoarthritis

OA causes the knee to become increasingly painful and tender. Inflammation and loss of cartilage also lead to stiffness, joint deformity, and restricted movements. You may feel or hear creaking and cracking as you move and the joint may become swollen due to a build up of fluid (effusion). Walking awkwardly causes ligaments and muscles to ache, and joint pain may keep you awake at night. The muscles around affected joints may become weak and wasted from lack of use.

occurs is largely irreversible. X-ray studies involving people aged 45 or over show that around 15% of men and 24% of women have evidence of OA within their knee joints. It is more common in women, in people who are overweight, and in joints damaged by sports injuries and accidents.

WHEN IS KNEE REPLACEMENT NECESSARY?

Meniscectomy

Damage to the cartilage disks (menisci) in the knee joints predisposes to OA to the extent that nearly 50% of people undergoing open knee surgery to remove all or part of a damaged meniscus (meniscectomy) develop OA of the knee within 21 years after surgery.

Knee replacement surgery is usually performed when osteoarthritis within the joint causes persistent pain, which may keep you awake at night, deformity, or immobility that interferes with daily life. Joint replacement aims to remove the affected parts of the joint and insert artificial components to stop pain and improve mobility.

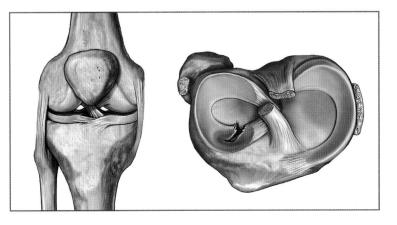

RIGHT The anatomy of the right knee joint (left) revealing a torn meniscus injury viewed from above (right).

Knee Replacement
Step-by-step

Partial or total knee replacement

You may have a partial (unicompartmental) knee replacement, involving the end of just one bone (tibia or femur) or a total knee replacement, in which the ends of both bones (and often the patella) are renewed. Total knee replacement is by far the most common, accounting for over 90% of cases. The artificial joint that is inserted is known as a prosthesis (plural prostheses). For a total knee replacement, the prosthesis consists of a two, polished, metal alloy components (usually based on titanium or cobalt/chromium) which replace the ends of the long bones, and a high-density plastic liner (polyethylene) which sits on the tibia to separate the two. Sometimes, the back of the patella is also resurfaced with plastic. Most prostheses are held in place with a "bone cement" such as polymethylmethacrylate, which "dries" quickly. Some prostheses are cementless, and specially textured or coated to encourage new bone to grow in and secure them. Screws or pegs are used to stabilize them until bone growth occurs. These require a longer healing time than cemented joints. Sometimes, a hybrid technique is used, in which the femoral component is inserted without cement, but the tibial and patellar components are cemented in.

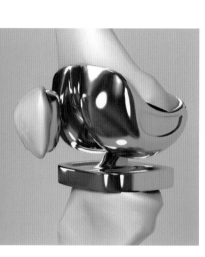

ABOVE A metal, artificial knee replacement showing how the prosthesis fits over the prepared bone ends.

❶ Once the patient is asleep, the anesthesiologist injects a muscle relaxant drug to reduce tension in the leg muscles. A tight tourniquet is applied to the thigh to stop blood flow to the leg. The surgeon makes an incision down the front of the knee that is from 8 in to 12 in (20 cm to 30 cm) long, depending on whether you are having a partial or total knee replacement. The incision may be made with the knee straight or flexed, depending on surgeon preference. The quadriceps muscle may be cut enough to allow the kneecap to be turned over or pulled to one side to expose the knee joint. The joint capsule is then opened (arthrotomy).

RIGHT Marks made on the skin before the initial incision will help the surgon when closing the wound.

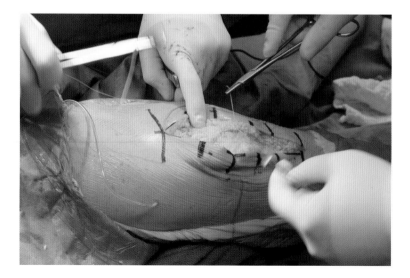

RIGHT The orthopedic surgeon is using an oscillating saw to prepare the surface of the tibia bone for the replacement knee.

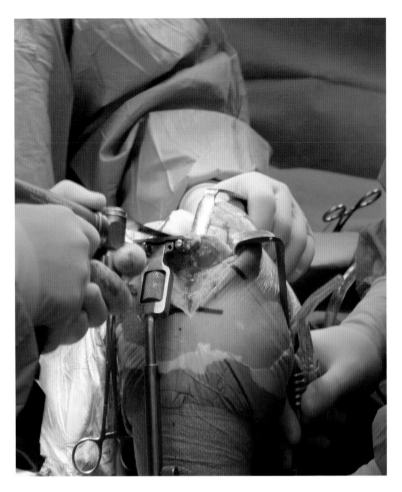

BELOW Full protective clothing is worn during a knee replacement as tiny fragments of bone are thrown up by the electric saw.

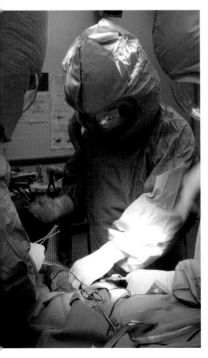

❷ With the knee flexed to 90 degrees, retractors are used to hold back and protect the soft tissues and the kneecap. The damaged lower surface of the femur is removed with a special electric saw and shaped, using a special cutting guide, to fit the new, artificial femoral component. Using a template, holes are drilled up into the lower end of the cut femur to locate the new prosthesis.

❸ The damaged surface of the tibia is removed and shaped to fit the new, artificial tibial component *(see above)*. A hole is drilled down into the top of the prepared tibia to accept a peg on the base plate. Some components require the tibia to be shaped to accept a longer stem.

Cutting bone

The surgical team wear full protective clothing to avoid contact with fine bone fragments thrown up by the saw *(see left)*. The saw is cooled using constant irrigation — if it is allowed to heat bone above 113 °F (45 °C) for more than one minute, long-term bone damage can occur.

ENSURING A SMOOTHLY FUNCTIONING JOINT

❹ If the back of the kneecap is rough or damaged, it must be resurfaced to ensure smooth functioning of the new joint. With the knee straightened, the patella is partially dissected and its thickness assessed. The back of the patella is then shaved off — usually a depth of around 0.3 in (8 mm) is removed — and planed smooth. Shallow holes are then drilled into the kneecap to locate the new plastic component, which is pushed into place using a special clamp.

❺ The new tibial and femoral components are then temporarily positioned, and the alignment and stability of the joint is checked both when the knee is straight and when bent. Any necessary adjustments are made to fine-tune the fit. When the surgeon is happy with the alignment, the metal components are refitted using bone cement *(see below)*. Bone screws may be used to further stabilize the metal components. The plastic liner is then pushed into position between the new metal ends of the bones and it clips into place.

❻ The tourniquet is let down and the knee taken through the full range of movement to check all is well. The joint is thoroughly cleansed of bone chips and cement which might cause excessive wear on the new

BELOW Gluing the components of the new joint in place.

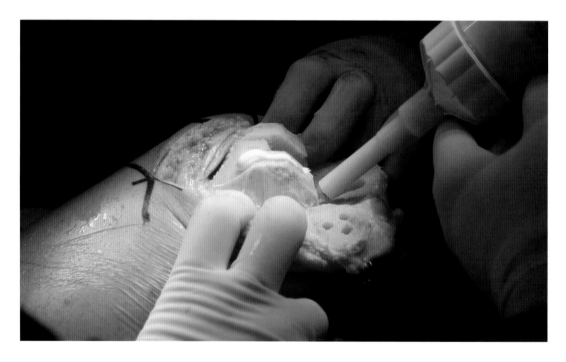

Mini-incision total knee replacement

The new mini-incision technique for total knee replacement can reduce recovery time following surgery. Smaller instruments are used, and the kneecap is slid to the side with minimal cutting of the quadriceps thigh muscle. This requires an incision that is only 4 to 5 in (10 to 13 cm) long.

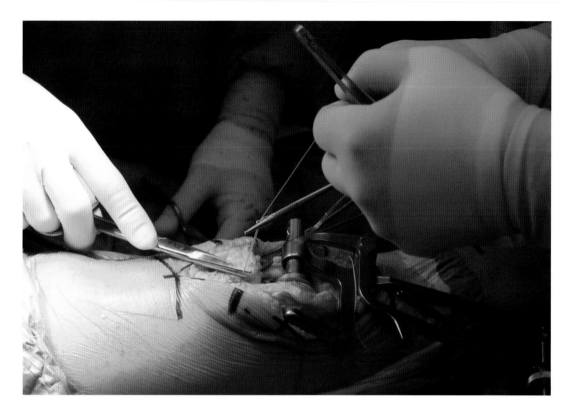

ABOVE A patellar clamp holds
the new lining in place against
the kneecap.

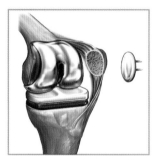

ABOVE A diagram showing where
the patellar button component
fits on the back of the knee bone.

joint. The joint capsule is then closed, and the skin wound repaired
with stitches or clips. A tight dressing is applied to help reduce
swelling. A drain may be left in place to prevent fluid building up
around the knee. This is removed after one or two days. If absorbable
stitches are used, these usually dissolve and disappear within seven to
ten days. Non-absorbable sutures and clips are removed after seven to
ten days of recuperation.

Antibiotics are given during and after surgery to help reduce
chances of infection of the wound or joint.

The Food and Drug Administration (FDA) is planning to create a
national joint orthopedic device register to follow up the safety,
durability, and effectiveness of different joint replacement devices and
procedures. At some stage you may be asked to consent to your name
being placed on the register if you have a joint implant.

Gender specific prostheses

Traditional knee prostheses are "unisex." Research
suggests that good implant fit depends on shape as
well as size, and knee joints specifically designed
for women are now available. These more closely
reflect the shape of a female knee — the femur
component has a thinner profile, and a narrower,
more contoured shape. This reduces bulkiness and,
as the implant does not overhang the bone and press
on surrounding ligaments and tendons, reduces
post-operative pain. It also allows for the different
alignment between the hip and knee that occurs in
women, so permitting a more natural movement.

KNEE REPLACEMENT
QUESTIONS & ANSWERS

What are the benefits?

Knee replacement relieves pain and restores good joint movement for nine out of ten people. The artificial knee usually lasts ten to 20 years before it needs to be replaced. New designs, materials, and techniques mean that replacement joints are lasting longer. Maintaining a sensible level of activity, and a healthy weight helps the joint last longer, too.

What are the risks?

As well as the general risks associated with surgery and general anesthesia *(see pages 10–11)*, there is an increased risk of blood clots in the leg (deep vein thrombosis or DVT). This is reduced by early mobilization, compression stockings, using an intermittent compression pump during and after surgery, and with blood-thinning medication. The knee may feel sore and remain swollen for up to a year. The skin around the scar may feel numb for many months and occasionally long-term. Excessive scar tissue formation may restrict movements, requiring surgery to correct the problem. The new joint may become loose or unstable, so you need a revision operation. X-ray checks at least every five years can detect early signs of loosening.

Are there any alternatives?

Knee pain and mobility may be improved with physical aids (walking sticks, crutches), physiotherapy, exercises, and analgesic medicines such as acetaminophen and/or non-steroidal anti-inflammatory drugs. Soft knee braces and shoe modifications (custom-made foot orthotics) also help. An injection of a corticosteroid drug into the knee may reduce pain and inflammation. Needle lavage (the washing out of a joint with saline) can remove loose bodies causing pain, such as bone or cartilage fragments. Glucosamine sulfate, chondroitin sulfate, and MSM (methylsulfonylmethane) supplements can reduce pain and may slow the progression of knee osteoarthritis. Cartilage grafting may prove possible for a knee with limited cartilage loss in one area.

What can I do to prepare?

Be as fit and healthy as possible. If you smoke, do your utmost to stop as smoking increases the risk of complications such as wound infection and blood clots. Losing excess weight reduces the compressive force

Excess weight increases joint damage

Every 1 lb (0.45 kg) increase in weight increases the overall force across your knee joints when walking or standing by 2 lb to 3 lb (0.9 kg to 1.4 kg). So, if you are 10 lb (4.5 kg) overweight, the force on your knees increases by up to 30 lb (13.5 kg). Looked at the other way round, losing 10 lb in weight (4.5 kg) can reduce the load on your knees by as much as 30 lb (13.5 kg).

on your joints, as well as reducing inflammation. The American Academy of Orthopedic Surgeons recommends that patients who are overweight, with a body mass index (BMI) of greater than 25 should lose a minimum of 5% body weight, and take up low-impact aerobic exercise to improve fitness.

What if I don't have the operation?

Your knee is likely to become increasingly painful and stiff, as osteoarthritis is a progressive disease in which low-grade inflammation causes continued damage.

What happens during the recovery period?

Pain relief helps to reduce discomfort as the anesthetic wears off. You may have a compression pump attached to your lower legs which inflates intermittently to encourage blood flow and reduce the risk of a blood clot (DVT). You may also have a compression stocking on the

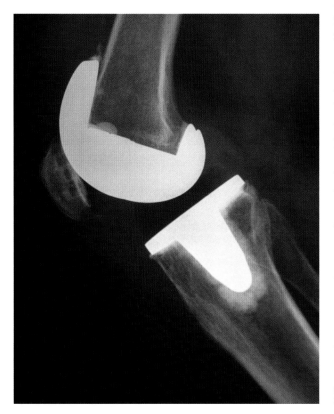

leg that was not operated on, and may receive injections of an anti-clotting medicine called heparin.

Physiotherapy usually starts the day after surgery, as regular daily exercises are vital for a rapid recovery and return to normal mobility. You can go home once you can get in and out of bed by yourself, bend your knee to approximately 90 degrees, straighten your knee fully, and safely walk with the aid of sticks or crutches both on the flat and up and down a few stairs. You will usually wear compression stockings for several weeks, and be advised to rest with your leg raised, and your knee supported, to reduce swelling of the ankles. Applying an ice pack for 15 minutes also helps to reduce swelling. You can usually return to work within six to eight weeks.

LEFT X-ray of a total knee replacement. This is a lateral view of the left knee.

HYSTERECTOMY

Hysterectomy means the surgical removal of the uterus, or womb. In some cases, the ovaries are also removed (oophorectomy) which will trigger a premature menopause. Usually, a surgeon tries to conserve at least one ovary in premenopausal women to prevent this, although estrogen replacement therapy can offset hot flashes and other symptoms if you are able to take it. If both the ovaries and Fallopian tubes (down which eggs travel from the ovaries to the womb) are also excised, the operation is known as a hysterectomy and bilateral salpingo-oophorectomy.

WHY A HYSTERECTOMY MAY BE NECESSARY

There are several gynecological reasons why a woman may be advised to have a hysterectomy, assuming that her family is complete. Where possible, however, other medical or surgical treatments are used instead, as most women prefer to keep their uterus and ovaries unless they are experiencing serious health problems. A common reason for requesting a hysterectomy is heavy, painful periods (menorrhagia) which can last for ten days or longer, with flooding and sometimes clots. This tends to occur in later life, when an egg fails to develop during a menstrual cycle. As a result, the womb lining continues to plump up and become thicker than normal, causing a heavier period. Another cause of heavy, painful periods is fibroids, in which muscular "knots" form in the uterine wall. If these are large and multiple, the uterus may become bulky causing considerable distension and pain, as well as heavy periods.

Hysterectomy may also be needed to treat endometriosis, in which endometrial (womb lining) cells develop outside the uterine cavity. Deposits may form on the surface of the uterus, within the uterine muscle tissue (adenomyosis), or on the surface of the ovaries. The cells involved respond to the hormonal menstrual cycle and may bleed into surrounding tissues at the time of menstruation, causing inflammation. Fluid-filled cysts (vesicles) and solid nodules may develop, especially on the ovaries, where large, chocolate-colored cysts can develop. Symptoms include persistent pain, which can be severe, especially around the time of menstruation.

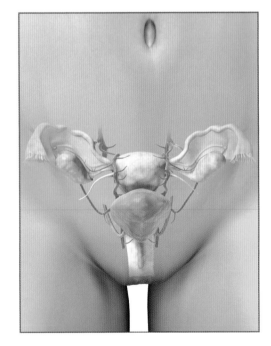

BELOW Female reproductive system showing healthy Fallopian tubes and uterus.

HYSTERECTOMY AT A GLANCE

• *Can it be done as an outpatient?* No. Admission to hospital is necessary.

• *Do I need a general anesthetic?* Usually, yes.

• *What special tests are needed?* None, usually. The decision to have a hysterectomy is usually made on the basis of troublesome symptoms that have not responded to other suitable treatments.

• *How long does the surgery take?* A total abdominal hysterectomy takes around one hour to complete. A laparoscopically assisted vaginal hysterectomy takes around two hours. A vaginal hysterectomy takes around 80 minutes. The larger the size of the womb, the longer the operation usually takes.

• *What is the mortality rate?* Less than one in 1000 (0.08%).

• *How long will I be in hospital?* Patients usually stay in hospital for two to five days, but it depends on the reason why the hysterectomy was performed. Women who are having an abdominal hysterectomy, those having their ovaries removed, and those aged 85 and older tend to stay in longest.

• *How expensive is it?* 💲

• *How many are performed in the US each year?* Around 525,000 hysterectomies are performed in the US each year. Having reached a high of 640,000 operations per year in 2001, the figures are now falling with the introduction of techniques that remove just the womb lining *(see page 73)*. The number of women having one or both ovaries removed (oophorectomy) is around 65,000 per year.

In women who have had several pregnancies, weakness of the pelvic floor muscles may fail to support the uterus, so it starts to descend through the vagina. Known as uterine prolapse, this causes discomfort and dragging sensations. Hysterectomy is also used to treat a cancer affecting the upper reproductive tract (cervix, uterus, ovaries, Fallopian tube).

Occasionally, hysterectomy is needed as a last resort after delivery of a baby when catastrophic postpartum hemorrhage cannot be stopped any other way.

A total (or complete) abdominal hysterectomy removes the whole uterus, including the cervix, through a low abdominal incision. A partial (sub-total or supracervical) abdominal hysterectomy involves removing just the body of the uterus, leaving the cervix and vagina intact. A woman who has this type of hysterectomy must continue having routine cervical (Pap) smears as there is still a normal risk of developing cervical cancer in the future. Vaginal hysterectomy is gaining in popularity, as it has the advantage of no abdominal scar and a quicker post-operative recovery. The vagina can be tightened at the same time, if necessary.

Age statistics

Around half the number of women having a hysterectomy are under the age of 44. One in ten is over the age of 65 years, and one in 20 is 85 years or older.

Hysterectomy
Step-by-step

Hysterectomy with or without oophorectomy

In younger women, hysterectomy without oophorectomy (removal of the ovaries) is carried out where possible. In older women who are approaching the menopause, hysterectomy plus oophorectomy may be advised. The advantage of having the ovaries removed as the menopause approaches is that you will not develop ovarian cancer. It is estimated that 1 in 500 women whose ovaries are conserved will develop an ovarian malignancy.

Hysterectomy may be carried out as a vaginal or abdominal operation. Where possible, the vaginal route is used, to avoid an abdominal scar, but around two thirds of operations are still performed via an abdominal incision. This is especially likely where there are large fibroids, endometriosis, or the ovaries are to be removed. During a laparoscopically assisted vaginal hysterectomy, part of the operation is performed abdominally and part vaginally *(see page 71)*.

If you are having a total abdominal hysterectomy (TAH), the surgeon will try to use a bikini-line incision. Occasionally a vertical scar is necessary if the uterus is exceptionally bulky with large fibroids, if there is a large ovarian cyst, widespread adhesions (scar tissue, e.g. from previous pelvic surgery or inflammation), or if a malignancy is suspected. A vertical scar is also needed if the surgeon wishes to examine the upper abdominal cavity — for example, if endometriosis is present on the surface of the liver.

❶ The bladder is emptied and a catheter is left in place during the operation to help the surgeon easily identify the urethra (urinary tube leading from the bladder to the outside). The vagina is then painted inside with a blue-dyed antiseptic. These measures help make these structures more easily identifiable during the operation, both to assist with identifying anatomical landmarks and to avoid damage to these delicate structures.

BELOW Incision of skin and uterus during total abdominal hysterectomy. The second view (right) shows a larger laparotomy incision which is rarely used.

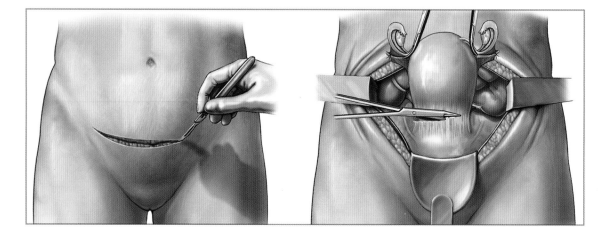

❷ The surgeon makes a horizontal incision along the lower abdomen. This is known as a Pfannenstiel or bikini incision. The wound is around 4 in to 5.5 in (10 cm to 14 cm) long, and is made using a hot "knife" that seals (cauterizes) the tissues to reduce bleeding. If the uterus is very bulky, due to large fibroids, a vertical incision may be used, which extends from just below the umbilicus (belly button) down to just above the pubic bone. Where inspection of the upper abdomen is needed, the midline incision may be extended around and above the umbilicus. Self-retaining retractors are used to hold the wound open, and the bowel is packed out of the way for protection, using warm, moist gauze packs.

BELOW Removal of an enlarged, bulky uterus.

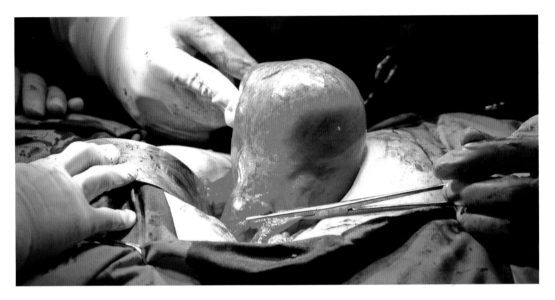

Vaginal hysterectomy

The uterus and ovaries can be removed via the vagina, as long as the womb is no larger than a 12 week pregnancy. In a standard vaginal hysterectomy, the uterus is entirely dissected out through incisions made in the top of the vagina. In a laparoscopically assisted vaginal hysterectomy, the initial parts of the operation are carried out abdominally, through tiny incisions, and the uterus is then removed vaginally. To do this, four or five small incisions are made in the lower abdomen and umbilicus. After inflating the abdomen with gas to improve access, and to help push the bowel out of the way, any pelvic adhesions are finely divided under direct visual control. The surgeon then manipulates the viewing device (laparoscope) and special long-handled surgical instruments through the abdominal incisions working to carefully free the womb. The ligaments supporting the uterus, and its main blood vessels, are clamped off, cut, and sealed. If the ovaries are to remain inside, the Fallopian tubes are clamped and cut away from the uterus, too. The uterus is then carefully cut away from its surroundings, and any bleeding points cauterized. The abdomen is then deflated and the hysterectomy completed by removing the uterus through the vagina. A circular incision is made around the cervix in the vaginal vault, and the uterus (with or without the fallopian tubes and ovaries) is removed by pulling it downward. The incision in the vault of the vagina is closed using a running stitch (to allow drainage) or an automatic stapling device.

REMOVING THE UTERUS

❸ The round ligaments (which hold the uterus in a tilted-forward position) are clamped, sealed, and cut. The uterus is then carefully dissected away from its surrounding structures, such as the broad ligament (a band of tissue suspending the uterus in the pelvis) and bladder. The bladder, which is attached to the lower segment of the uterus, is carefully "peeled" or cut away. If the ovaries and Fallopian tubes are to be left inside, these are also clamped, sealed, and cut *(see below)*.

❹ In a sub-total hysterectomy, the body of the uterus is sliced away just above the cervix, and removed, leaving the cervix and vagina intact. This procedure was initially popular as it was thought to reduce the chance of future sexual difficulties or urinary leakage. Recent research has found no evidence of differences in the outcomes between these two operations. Sub-total hysterectomy is a faster operation, however, with less blood loss and chance of infection, but women are more likely to have some ongoing regular menstrual bleeding as a result of some endometrial (womb lining) cells remaining. Regular cervical (Pap) smears are also needed.

RIGHT The bulky uterus is completely removed.

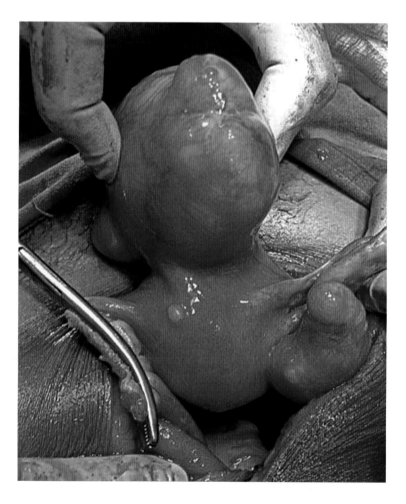

Endometrial ablation

Women with heavy periods but no fibroids may be suitable for endometrial ablation, in which the endometrium (womb lining) is destroyed using lasers, hot cutting wires (diathermy), radio-frequency waves, or heat sources. This leaves the muscular wall of the uterus intact and is a safer, less invasive alternative to hysterectomy. If the entire thickness of the endometrium is destroyed, no further menstrual bleeding will occur. Often, however, small areas of endometrial tissue are left behind, and around 70% of women experience light monthly bleeds. One in five women may require a repeat procedure to reduce blood loss within two years. Like hysterectomy, the procedure should only be performed in women who do not wish for further pregnancies.

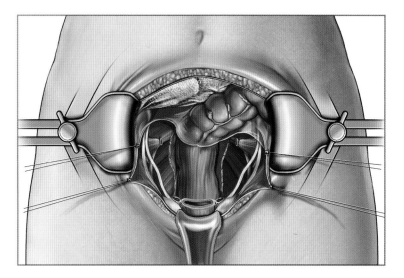

RIGHT The pelvis after removal of the uterus.

5 A total hysterectomy removes the cervix meaning there is no risk of developing future cervical cancer. This is something to discuss with your doctor — some women prefer to retain as much of their reproductive system as possible, including their cervix. During a total abdominal hysterectomy, the whole uterus is removed by clamping and cutting the uterine blood vessels, and ligaments at the base of the uterus. The body of the uterus is then pulled upward, cut away from the vagina, and removed.

6 The edges of the vagina are picked up with four clamps and the edges are oversewn and stitched into place, often leaving the vaginal cuff open. The upper opening to the vagina is then covered and protected by sewing together the cut peritoneal membrane that lines the pelvic and abdominal cavities. Leaving the vaginal vault open in this way to heal naturally over the next few weeks has been shown to dramatically reduce the risk of the patient developing a post-operative pelvic abscess.

HYSTERECTOMY
QUESTIONS & ANSWERS

What are the benefits?

A hysterectomy relieves you of further menstrual problems such as heavy bleeding or cyclical cramping pains. It also means that you no longer have to consider the use of contraceptive measures for the prevention of pregnancy (however, this procedure offers no protection against sexually transmitted infections).

What are the risks?

As well as the general risks associated with surgery and general anesthesia *(see pages 10–11)*, there is a risk of developing an infection in the pelvis which may result in a pelvic abscess. Antibiotics are given to help prevent this. Leaving the top of the vagina open, to heal on its own, rather than sealing it closed, also helps to reduce this risk. Occasionally, damage to other abdominal organs, such as the intestines, bladder, or ureters (urinary tubes leading from the kidneys to the bladder) may occur, which may need further surgery to repair.

If both ovaries are removed, menopausal symptoms will start immediately, and may be severe due to the sudden (rather than gradual) fall in estrogen levels. Where possible, this is counteracted with estrogen replacement therapy, but this is not always possible if you have an estrogen-dependent condition (e.g. endometriosis, some cancers). Where the ovaries are left in place, there is evidence that the menopause may occur three years earlier than normal. Where only one ovary is left in place, menopause may occur four years earlier than normal. This may relate to changes in blood flow to the ovaries as a result of hysterectomy.

Are there any alternatives?

Heavy menstrual bleeding may be reduced with hormonal drugs, blood clotting agents (e.g. tranexamic acid), or non-steroidal anti-inflammatory drugs (NSAIDs). Bleeding can be reduced by having the levonorgestrel-impregnated intrauterine system (Mirena IUS) fitted.

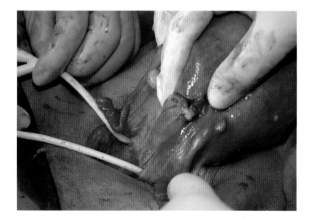

BELOW Fibroids being removed surgically (myomectomy).

This is a method of contraception that can significantly reduce menstrual blood loss. Bleeding may be increased initially, during the first three months after fitting, however.

Techniques are now available to remove or destroy the womb lining (endometrium) while keeping the uterine muscular wall intact. These can stop, or significantly reduce, menstrual flow. These avoid the physical and psychological traumas of a major operation and mean that total hysterectomy is likely to become less common in future *(see page 73)*.

Fibroids may be removed surgically (myomectomy) *(see opposite)*, destroyed by laser, or caused to shrink by reducing their blood supply (uterine artery embolization). A new treatment, called magnetic resonance guided focused ultrasound (MRgFUS) uses ultrasound waves to heat fibroids and destroy them.

Endometriosis may be treated with hormonal drugs (gonadotrophins) that produce a temporary menopause.

What can I do to prepare?

As well as ensuring that you are as fit as possible by losing any excess weight, and stopping smoking, it is important to prepare emotionally for the operation. Many women feel a great sense of loss and sadness following a hysterectomy, as they can no longer have a pregnancy. Even if your family is complete, and you may not think this will be a problem, having the choice taken away from you can be surprisingly upsetting. Talk to your doctor, and other women who have had a hysterectomy, if you can. If you are not certain you really want to have a hysterectomy, ask your doctor to help you explore all the other options available to you.

What if I don't have the operation?

If you don't have a hysterectomy, other alternative procedures or drugs may help to control your symptoms. A hysterectomy may eventually become necessary if you experience ongoing gynecological problems, however.

What happens during the recovery period?

You may still have a urinary catheter in place after the operation, but this is often not necessary. You are encouraged to start walking around on the day after surgery to reduce the risk of blood clots in the leg veins. The average hospital stay for TAH is around four days, but only two days for laparoscopically assisted vaginal hysterectomy. Recovery is similarly quicker with the latter operation, although the risk of complications is higher. Full recovery generally takes six to eight weeks for TAH, five weeks for vaginal hysterectomy, and three weeks for laparoscopic hysterectomy.

You may notice a brown-red discharge from the vagina for around a month after surgery. You can usually return to work five to six weeks after the operation. During the first few months after surgery, avoid lifting anything heavy, such as shopping bags and small children.

Resuming sexual intercourse

You can usually resume sexual intercourse four to six weeks after the operation, after having an internal examination to ensure full healing has occurred. You may notice vaginal dryness after the operation due to the loss of normal cervical discharge. Using a lubricant will help to overcome problems during sex.

HIP REPLACEMENT

Hip replacement is one of the most common orthopedic procedures in the US. The hip is a ball-and-socket joint formed between the head of the thigh bone (femur) which forms the ball, and a cup-shaped depression (acetabulum) in the pelvis, which forms the socket. Hip replacement may be needed when the joint becomes stiff and painful from a degenerative disease, such as osteoarthritis. Other indications include severe fracture after an accident or fall, loss of blood supply to the head of the femur (which dies and crumbles away), infection of the bone, and developmental abnormalities of the hip.

HOW DOES OSTEOARTHRITIS AFFECT THE HIP JOINT?

Osteoarthritis causes the hip joint to become increasingly painful. This is partly because inflammation stimulates the growth of new blood vessels and sensory nerve endings into the joint, and partly because low-grade inflammation causes the nerves to become more sensitive. Although traditionally thought of as a wear-and-tear disease, osteoarthritis is now believed to result from the active repair of damaged joints. Less new cartilage is made to replace that which has broken down, however, so repair is incomplete. Cartilage becomes weaker, stiffer, and less able to withstand compressive forces. As a result, the articular cartilage protecting the bone ends becomes pitted, cracked, and starts to flake away. Synovial fluid leaks into the underlying bone, causing mild inflammation, bone thickening, and the formation of small cysts and bony outgrowths known as osteophytes.

Risk factors

• People with previous hip injury are over four times more likely to have osteoarthritis of the hip and to need a hip replacement than those without previous hip injury. The average time to develop osteoarthritis of the hip following a fracture dislocation is seven years.

• Being overweight is a clear risk factor for OA in weight-bearing joints, such as the hip. Obesity increases the chance that you will need a hip replacement by 70% compared with those of normal weight. Being overweight early in life appears to increase the risk further, as your joints are subjected to the harmful effects of excess weight for longer.

HIP REPLACEMENT AT A GLANCE

- **Can it be done as an outpatient?** No. Admission to hospital is necessary.

- **Do I need a general anesthetic?** Usually, yes. An alternative is to have a spinal-epidural local anesthetic which both numbs and relaxes you from the waist down, so you stay awake during the operation *(see page 8)*. This may be suggested for people who are less likely to tolerate a general anesthetic — perhaps because of lung disease. There is a lot of pulling and pushing during surgery, however, and a general anesthetic is the best option.

- **What special tests are needed?** Damage to the hip can be assessed by X-ray. A CT, MRI, or bone scan may be needed to determine the condition of your bones and soft tissues, and to help your orthopedic surgeon plan the operation. Blood tests can help to diagnose some types of joint inflammation, such as rheumatoid arthritis.

- **How long does the surgery take?** Traditional hip replacement operations take 45 to 60 minutes. Newer, less invasive techniques take longer, at between one and two hours.

- **What is the mortality rate?** Less than one in 100 (0.9%).

- **How long will I be in hospital?** Traditionally, people having a hip replacement stayed in hospital for eight to 12 days. Newer procedures mean that many patients are able to start walking within hours of surgery, and can therefore go home earlier. Some people, who are otherwise fit and well, can even go home the day after surgery. The average hospital stay is four to five days.

- **How expensive is it?** $ $

- **How many are performed in the US each year?** Around 370,000 operations are performed in the US each year. Hip replacements are more common in women, who account for 60% of operations. Most hip replacements occur in people over the age of 55. Two thirds are aged 65 and over.

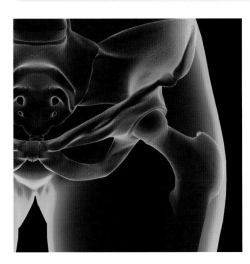

Inflammation, loss of cartilage, and osteophyte formation lead to joint deformity, stiffness, and restricted movements. You may feel or hear creaking and cracking as you move. Walking awkwardly causes ligaments and muscles to ache, and joint pain may keep you awake at night. The muscles around affected joints may become weak and wasted from lack of use.

A hip replacement operation is usually recommended once hip pain and stiffness interfere with your quality of life, affect your ability to sleep, or mean that you experience difficulty walking very far.

LEFT A diagram showing osteoarthrosis of the hip joint.

Joint replacement register

The FDA (Food and Drug Administration) is planning to create a national joint orthopedic device register to follow up the safety, durability, and effectiveness of different joint replacement devices and procedures. At some stage you may be asked to consent to your name being placed on the register if you have a joint implant.

HIP REPLACEMENT
STEP-BY-STEP

TOTAL OR PARTIAL HIP REPLACEMENT

In a partial hip replacement, just the head of the femur (ball) or, sometimes, just the acetabulum (socket) is replaced. During a total hip replacement, both the damaged ball and socket are removed and replaced with artificial structures. Total hip replacement is by far the most common, accounting for over 90% of cases.

The artificial joint that is inserted is known as a prosthesis (plural prostheses). The new socket is usually made from high-density plastic (polyethylene), metal (e.g. cobalt chrome), or ceramic, while the femoral component is made from a strong, polished, stainless metal or ceramic, whose stem is slotted down the center of the femur. Some components are fixed in place with a strong bone cement, such as polymethyl-methacrylate, which "dries" quickly. Others are designed as cementless and are specially textured or coated to encourage new bone to grow in and secure them. Screws may be used to stabilize them until bone growth occurs. Cementless joints require a longer healing time than cemented joints. Sometimes, a hybrid technique is used, in which the femoral component is cemented in, but the socket is non-cemented. Cementless components are used most often in young, active people with strong bones.

The hip joint is deeply placed. It can be accessed through frontal (anterior), rear (posterior), and side (lateral) approaches. For a total hip replacement, a front-at-the-side (anterolateral) approach is used where possible, in which the incision extends from the top of the hip bone, down the side of the upper femur. This approach does not involve cutting the abductor muscles needed to move the leg away from the body.

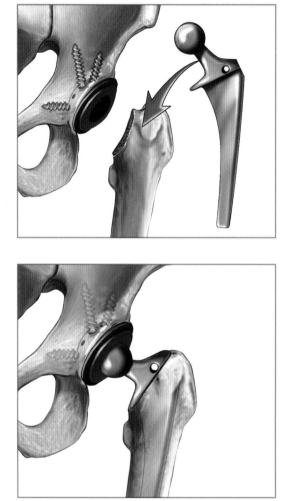

ABOVE A hip replacement prosthesis, showing the details of the femoral component (top) and with both the acetabular component and the femoral component in place (above).

❶ Once the patient is asleep, the anesthesiologist injects a muscle relaxant drug to reduce tension in the leg muscles. An anterolateral incision is made that extends from the top of the hip bone at the front (anterior, superior iliac spine) down toward the top of the shaft of the femur *(see opposite)*. The cut is usually between 6 in and 12 in (15 cm and 30 cm) long, depending on whether you are having a partial or total hip replacement. The surgeon then cuts along the line between a buttock muscle (gluteus medius) and another muscle (tensor fascia lata) to split them apart. The gluteus medius muscle is pulled backward, and the tendon of the underlying, smaller buttock muscle (gluteus minimus) is cut to expose the joint capsule.

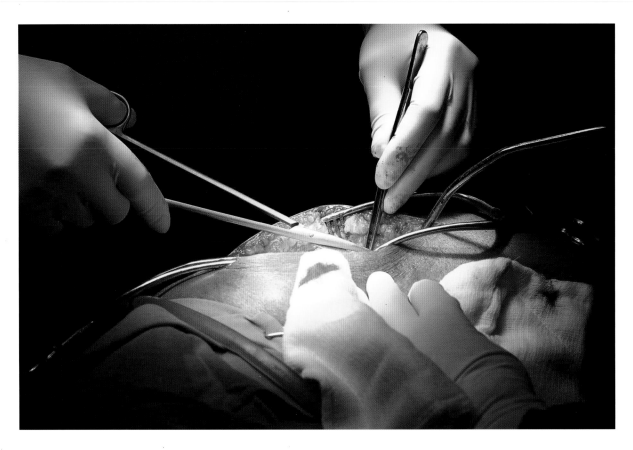

ABOVE The surgeon exposes the hip joint with a pair of Mayo scissors. These are heavy duty dissecting scissors with narrow blades.

❷ The surgeon takes a baseline measurement of the length of the leg. He or she then cuts into the hip joint capsule and literally pulls the ball and socket joint apart to dislocate the hip and expose the bone surfaces. The damaged head of the femur is removed by cutting the bone with a special electric saw. The cut is made at an angle of approximately 45 degrees to the shaft of the femur.

Minimally invasive procedures

New minimally invasive operations have been developed which involve making shorter (3 in to 6 in / 8 cm to 15 cm) single incisions. A "2-Incision" approach has also been developed for a cementless prosthesis. This involves making two small cuts, 1.5 in to 2 in (4 cm to 5 cm) in length, on either side of the hip joint. Then, rather than cutting leg and hip muscles to get at the joint, the muscles are simply moved to one side. This allows patients to mobilize more quickly after the operation. Minimally invasive procedures use specially designed instruments to operate through the smaller opening(s). X-ray guidance may be needed and it

takes longer to perform this surgery than with a traditional hip replacement. The benefits, however, include a shorter hospital stay, smaller scars, reduced blood loss, faster and less painful rehabilitation, and the possibility of a quicker return to work and normal daily life. Minimally invasive procedures are ideal for young, slim, otherwise healthy people who are likely to make a rapid recovery. Those not suitable for these procedures include people with abnormal anatomy from old congenital dislocation of the hip or a deformed fracture, and people with significant bone thinning (osteoporosis).

PREPARING THE HIP SOCKET

❸ The damaged surface of the hip socket (acetabulum) is removed and shaped to fit the new, artificial component. A new, cup-shaped implant is then pressed into the bone and may be secured with screws *(see below and below left)*. A smooth, plastic surface is then inserted which will allow the new joint to move freely.

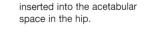

RIGHT An acetabular shell is inserted into the acetabular space in the hip.

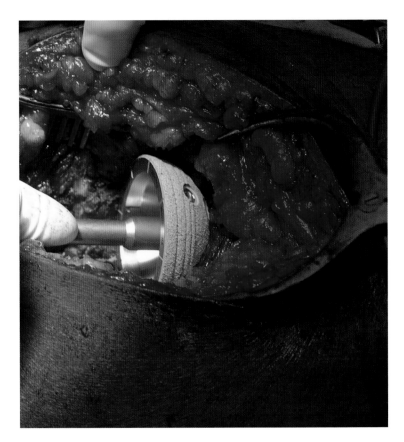

❹ The sawn-off head of the femur is prepared by exposing and reaming out the upper part of the femoral canal which runs down the middle of the femoral shaft *(see opposite above)*. This creates a hollow into which the new femoral prosthesis is inserted to a depth of about 6 in (15 cm). With a temporary prosthesis in place, the surgeon puts the joint back together to check the fit and leg length. If necessary, a longer or shorter final prosthesis can be used to ensure the final leg length is the same after the operation as it was before.

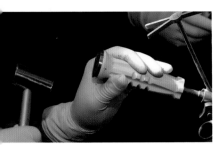

ABOVE The surgeon taps the acetabular shell into position using an impactor handle.

Porous metal

Scientists have developed a porous metal surface for cementless prostheses that resembles the honeycomb structure of bone. This encourages rapid and extensive infiltration with natural bone to hold the new, artificial component strongly in place.

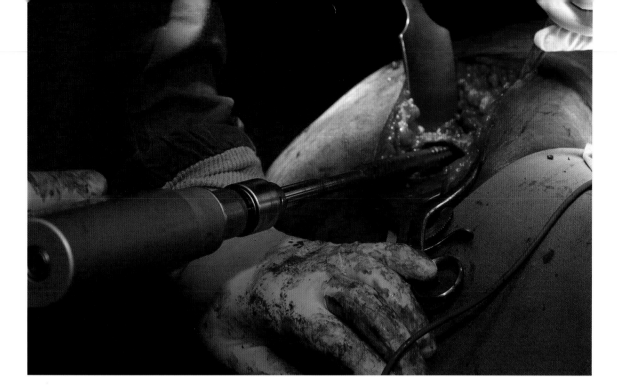

ABOVE Preparing the femoral canal with a drill.

BELOW Cleaning the newly sealed hip replacement wound.

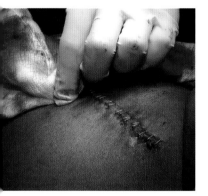

❺ Depending on the design of the prosthesis, the stem of the implant is either fixed in place with bone cement, or implanted and firmly impacted without cement. A metal ball is then placed on the top of the stem to act as the femoral head, and this is guided into place within the new socket.

❻ The hip joint is taken through the full range of movement to check all is well. The joint is thoroughly cleansed of bone chips and cement which might cause excessive wear on the new joint. The joint capsule is then closed, and the skin wound repaired with stitches or clips. A drain may be left in place to prevent fluid building up around the knee. This is removed after one or two days. If absorbable stitches are used, these usually dissolve and disappear within seven to ten days. Non-absorbable sutures and clips are removed after seven to ten days.

Antibiotics are given during and after surgery to help reduce the risk of infection of the wound or joint.

Personal tailoring

It is now possible to have a hip replacement prosthesis personally tailored to your individual measurements. Your hip is scanned using computerized tomography and a computer builds a 3D image of the required prosthesis. The new hip is then custom-made by a computerized milling machine that fashions it from titanium. The prosthesis is designed to fit tightly in place, without the need for cement. The two surfaces of the artificial joint are covered with a hard-wearing ceramic liner. Once the artificial joint is inserted, your own bone is stimulated to grow into the prosthesis to hold it in place. Where necessary, a hybrid operation can be carried out in which just one of the components — either the ball or socket — is cemented in place while the other part remains cementless.

HIP REPLACEMENT
QUESTIONS & ANSWERS

What are the benefits?

Hip replacement relieves pain and restores good joint movement for nine out of ten people. The artificial hip usually lasts ten to 15 years before it needs to be replaced. New designs, materials, and techniques mean replacement joints are lasting longer. Maintaining a sensible level of activity, and a healthy weight helps the joint last longer, too.

What are the risks?

As well as the general risks associated with surgery and general anesthesia *(see pages 10–11)*, a total hip replacement carries the risk of complications such as infection and deep vein blood clots. With newer procedures, however, pain is reduced, the risk of a blood clot is lessened (because less time is spent lying in bed), and the risk of picking up a wound infection in hospital is also less due to returning home more quickly. Occasionally, the joint becomes dislocated when the head of the femur comes out of the socket. This is most likely to happen if you have revision surgery (replacement of an old artificial hip). Sometimes, the leg is slightly longer or shorter than before, so you need to wear a raised shoe on the shorter side.

Are there any alternatives?

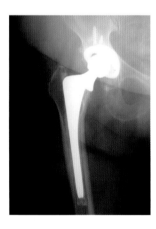

ABOVE An X-ray showing a total hip replacement that is secured with cement.

Hip pain and mobility may be improved with physical aids (walking sticks, crutches), physiotherapy, exercises, and analgesic medicines such as acetaminophen and/or non-steroidal anti-inflammatory drugs. Glucosamine sulfate, chondroitin sulfate, and MSM supplements can reduce pain and may slow the progression of hip osteoarthritis.

Hip-resurfacing arthroplasty can replace the damaged surfaces of the femoral head and acetabulum with metal parts to reduce pain and improve mobility. Less bone is removed than with a traditional hip replacement, making it easier to repeat the operation or to proceed to a total hip joint replacement in later life. Metal-on-metal hip resurfacing is best suited to people under the age of 55 who are a healthy weight.

The hip joint can also be fused to lock the bones into place, stabilizing the joint and relieving pain. This procedure is only performed on a weight-bearing joint such as the hip where replacement is not suitable, for example because of poor bone quality (osteoporosis) or abnormal anatomy from a congenital dislocation of the hip, a deformed fracture, or where previous joint replacement has failed.

What can I do to prepare?

Try to be as fit and healthy as possible before the operation, and lose some excess weight. If you smoke, do your utmost to stop to reduce your risk of deep vein blood clots and wound infection. Try to strengthen muscles in your upper body as well as your lower body. Assess your home, rearrange furniture for easy navigation.

What if I don't have the operation?

If you do not have the operation, it is likely that pain and immobility will slowly get worse.

What happens during the recovery period?

You may have a special pillow placed between your legs to hold the new hip joint still and help prevent dislocation. You may have a compression pump attached to your lower legs which inflates intermittently to encourage blood flow and reduce the risk of a blood clot (DVT or deep vein thrombosis). A compression stocking is usually fitted on the leg that was not operated on, and you may receive injections of an anti-clotting medicine called heparin.

Physiotherapy usually starts the day after surgery, as regular daily exercises are vital for a rapid recovery and return to normal mobility. You will be advised not to cross your legs, or twist your hip inward and outward during the first six weeks after surgery.

RIGHT A range of rasps used as femoral prostheses for total hip replacement operations.

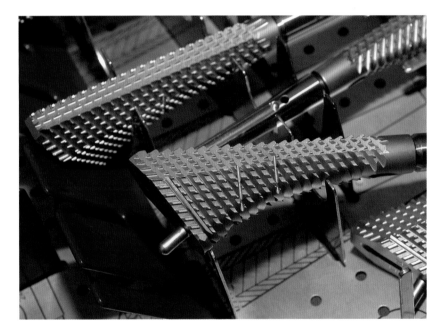

Lifestyle modifications

- Exercises are important to strengthen your muscles. As you recover, you will be advised when you can start swimming, walking, and golf. You must avoid high impact or contact sports, such as running, jumping, soccer, and basketball, however. You must also avoid activities that involve fast stopping and starting or twisting.
- You can usually return to work within six to eight weeks. If your job involves a lot of standing or lifting, you may need to take three months off work.
- You should not drive until your surgeon advises that you can — usually when you can perform an emergency stop without discomfort.
- Carry a medic alert card indicating you have an artificial joint if flying, in case an over-sensitive airport metal detector is activated by a metal prosthesis.

BREAST LUMPECTOMY/ MASTECTOMY

Lumpectomy and total mastectomy are surgical procedures used in the treatment of breast cancer. Lumpectomy removes just the breast lump, while mastectomy removes the whole breast and associated tissues, such as lymph nodes.

WHO GETS BREAST CANCER?

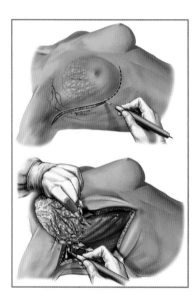

ABOVE Diagram of a mastectomy to remove cancerous breast tissue and lymph nodes.

Around 182,000 women are diagnosed with breast cancer in the United States each year, along with 1700 men. It affects one in eight women at some stage of their life, making it the most common female cancer.

Although most women experiencing breast cancer will not have a family history of the condition, breast cancer does run in some families. This is especially likely if a close relative (mother, sister, or daughter) was diagnosed before the age of 50 years, or if it has affected several generations in your family. The most likely cause of this increased risk is through inheriting a breast cancer gene.

Other women who may be at increased risk of breast cancer include those who:
• Started their periods aged 12 or younger.
• Have not had children.
• Have their first child after the age of 30.
• Have a late menopause after age 55.
• Use hormone replacement therapy (estrogen plus progestin) after the menopause.
• Are overweight or obese after the menopause.

These factors increase your lifetime exposure to the female hormone, estrogen. The number of women experiencing breast cancer fell by 10% between 2000 and 2004, which is thought to be partly due to reduced use of hormone replacement therapy.

Other factors that are linked with an increased risk of breast cancer include increasing age, drinking alcohol regularly, smoking cigarettes,

Screening mammography

Screening mammography uses X-rays to take images of the breasts from two directions. This aims to detect breast changes that may be due to early breast cancer. These include irregular, speckled shadows, small or clustered areas of calcification, and tissue distortion. Screening is repeated at regular intervals, usually annually, to look for changes.

BREAST LUMPECTOMY/MASTECTOMY AT A GLANCE

- *Can it be done as an outpatient?* Breast biopsy and lumpectomy are often performed as an outpatient. Mastectomy requires inpatient care.

- *Do I need a general anesthetic?* Breast biopsy and lumpectomy may be performed under local anesthesia unless removal of armpit lymph nodes is planned. General anesthesia is needed for lumpectomy with lymph node dissection, and for total mastectomy.

- *What special tests are needed?* You may be offered a diagnostic mammogram (which takes more detailed images of abnormal areas than screening mammography) or ultrasound to investigate the lump. A fine needle may be inserted to collect fluid or cells for examination under a microscope, or a larger tissue sample may be taken under local anesthesia (core biopsy). Some women may have an immediate lumpectomy, without awaiting further tests, so the lump can be fully examined in the laboratory. A bone scan may be suggested to look for distant spread.

- *How long does the surgery take?* From one to three hours, or more, depending on the extent of lymph node dissection and whether or not reconstruction is carried out.

- *What is the mortality rate?* The mortality rate associated with mastectomy is low, ranging from less than 1% in otherwise well, young, healthy women to 2.5% in older women with more extensive disease.

- *How long will I be in hospital?* Biopsy and breast lumpectomy may be performed as a day case. Women who have a breast lumpectomy or mastectomy in hospital tend to stay for two to three days.

- *How expensive is it?* $ to $$ depending on the procedure.

- *How many are performed in the US each year?* Breast lump biopsy: Around 276,000 women have the procedure as an outpatient, and 4500 as an inpatient. Breast lumpectomy: 346,000 women have the procedure as an outpatient, and 14,000 as an inpatient. Around 63,000 mastectomy operations are performed annually. Between 100 and 150 men have a breast lump biopsied each year, and 660 men undergo mastectomy.

and eating a diet that is high in fat (especially animal fat) and low in fiber, fruit, and vegetables.

Breast feeding for longer than one year, physical activity, and eating a Mediterranean-style diet seem to protect against breast cancer.

HOW IS BREAST CANCER DETECTED?

Breast cancer is detected through screening mammography *(see page 84)* or by a woman detecting a lump, or thickening, in her breast or armpit. Other signs that may occur in breast cancer include nipple tenderness, discharge, or the nipple turning inward. Sometimes, part of the breast or nipple may become scaly, red, swollen, or pitted like an orange skin. The diagnosis is confirmed with a biopsy to examine cells under a microscope.

HOW IS BREAST CANCER TREATED?

If breast cancer is diagnosed, you and your oncologist need to decide, together, whether lumpectomy or mastectomy (with breast reconstruction where appropriate) is your best option for a cure. Follow up medical treatment such as radiotherapy, chemotherapy, or anti-estrogen therapy is usually needed.

LUMPECTOMY/MASTECTOMY
STEP-BY-STEP

TOTAL MASTECTOMY

A mastectomy is one of the most emotive operations that a woman can have. As screening often allows breast cancer to be detected at an early stage, your doctors will only recommend mastectomy if they think this offers you the best chance of a cure. Although surgeons try to use breast-sparing surgery where possible, there has been a trend back toward mastectomy because of the development of reconstruction techniques that provide a warm, soft, natural, new breast. Many women also feel more comfortable in the knowledge that the source of their cancer has been removed completely.

Total (or simple) mastectomy removes the entire breast but preserves the chest muscles and lymph nodes in the armpit. These nodes are, instead, sampled using a technique known as sentinel lymph node biopsy *(see page 89)*. Radical mastectomy removes the breast, overlying skin, chest muscles, and all the tissues in the armpit. Extended radical mastectomy also includes removal of lymph nodes in the chest. This operation is rarely performed.

BELOW A large swab is placed under the dissected portion of the breast to soak up any blood.

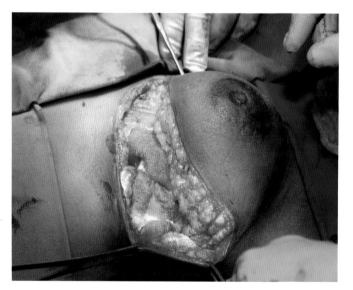

1 In a traditional mastectomy, the surgeon pulls the breast firmly downward and draws a straight line to define the upper incision. He then pulls the breast upward and draws a similar line to define the lower incision. The nipple, areola, and any previous biopsy scars are included in the area to be removed.

2 The surgeon cuts through the skin at the defined lines. He or she starts to make skin flaps by carefully dissecting between the breast tissue and the overlying layer of fat beneath the skin *(see left)*. Small bleeding points are sealed with heat (diathermy).

Skin-sparing mastectomy

An increasingly popular technique is the skin-sparing mastectomy, which removes the breast tissues through an incision around the nipple. This leaves an "envelope" of skin that can be used for immediate reconstruction, giving an even better cosmetic result. Other options are a nipple-sparing mastectomy that leaves the areola intact, or the total skin-sparing mastectomy that leaves all the skin, including the nipple and areola intact. These procedures are not suitable for everyone, however. They are particularly useful for women with a high risk of breast cancer who have chosen to undergo prophylactic bilateral mastectomy before cancer has developed.

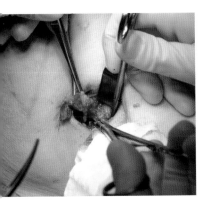

❸ The surgeon cuts through Cooper's ligaments, which suspend breast tissue from the overlying skin, and continues dissecting toward the breast bone (sternum) in the middle, the fold between the breast and the chest wall at the base (inframammary fold), the collar bone (clavicle) at the top, and the wing-shaped latissimus dorsi muscle at the side *(see below)*.

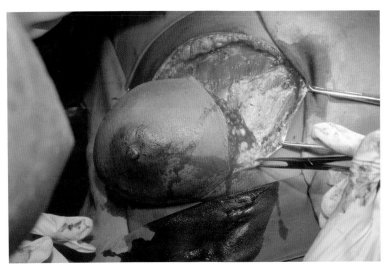

❹ For a simple mastectomy, the surgeon does not cut into the fat pad of the armpit. For a radical mastectomy, the surgeon now delves up into the armpit to remove all the fat and lymph nodes, taking care not to damage important nerves and blood vessels *(see below)*.

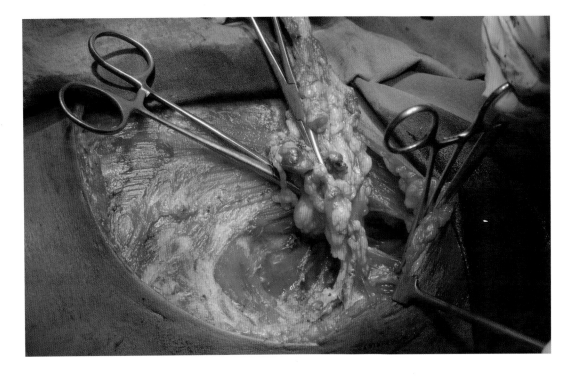

BREAST RECONSTRUCTION

❺ Where possible, immediate breast reconstruction is now performed. One option is to take a flap of skin and muscle from the rectus abdominis muscle. Known as a transverse rectus abdominis myocutaneous (TRAM) flap, it uses muscle, fat, and tissue from your midriff to reconstruct a realistic breast. An abdominal wall flap is fashioned from below the bikini line. It includes an orange-segment-shaped crescent of skin and its underlying fat, plus one of the two rectus abdominis muscles that run up and down the center of the abdomen. This tissue is either pivoted up (under the abdominal wall) through 180°, with the muscle still attached to its blood supply at the top (pedical method), or removed completely and reconnected to a blood supply in the armpit (free flap method). The free flap method requires microsurgery skills.

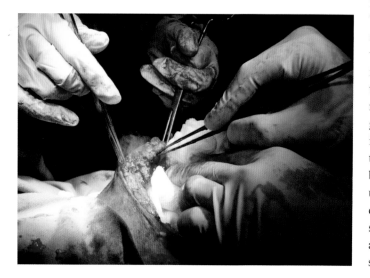

BELOW Surgeons performing a breast lumpectomy.

The pivotal method may leave a slight bump beneath the skin where the muscle is turned on itself. Synthetic material is used to replace the removed rectus muscle in the abdomen, and the gap in the lower abdominal wall is sewn up in a similar way to a tummy tuck, to leave a scar below the bikini line. A nipple is usually reconstructed at a later date. The opposite breast may be surgically lifted at the same time as the TRAM procedure to give a symmetrical result.

Lumpectomy

For women whose breast cancer is discovered while it is still small and in the early stages, breast-conserving surgery which removes just the lump is the most usual treatment. Known as lumpectomy, or wide local incision, the surgeon makes a long, curved incision directly over the lump. He or she then removes the breast lump plus an area of 0.2 in to 0.4 in (0.5 cm to 1 cm) of normal tissue around it *(see above)*. If the lump is very small, a wider margin of 0.8 in to 1.2 in (2 cm to 3 cm) is taken. The surgeon may also take samples of the underarm (axillary) lymph nodes through a separate incision. Removed tissues are sent for immediate "frozen" examination under a microscope to ensure that the cut edges are free from cancer cells. If the margins

are not clear, more tissue must be removed (in some cases, the surgeon may have to proceed to total mastectomy). After stopping any bleeding points, the incision is closed with an invisible, subcuticular stitch that will heal to leave minimal scarring. If sentinel lymph node sampling is planned *(see page 89)*, a separate incision is made in the hair-bearing skin of the armpit. After carefully identifying important nerves and blood vessels, muscle tissue is retracted out of the way and the fat and lymph nodes in the armpit are cut away.

Lumpectomy plus a course of radiotherapy (which destroys any cancer cells left in the breast) appears to be as effective as removal of the whole breast (mastectomy) for treating early cancer.

Sentinel lymph node biopsy

A less invasive method of lymph node sampling can be used for early breast cancer *(see page 87, top left)*. Known as sentinel lymph node biopsy, it aims to identify the sentinel lymph node, which is the first one to which cancer is likely to spread. The surgeon injects a harmless radioactive isotope (technetium-99m colloid) into the breast near the tumor, two hours before the operation. The tissues are massaged to reduce stinging and to encourage uptake into the lymphatics. Just before the biopsy, a blue dye is injected into the same place. The isotope and dye travel to the armpit in the lymph vessels, taking the same route through the body as a cancer cell might. The surgeon then uses a gamma probe to detect where the isotope has concentrated within the armpit, and cuts into this "hot spot." He or she then inspects the lymph nodes and removes those that show up as blue-green, or which have the highest isotope activity. These are sent for rapid analysis under a microscope while the surgeon proceeds to lumpectomy. If cancer cells are detected in the lymph nodes during their analysis, more extensive dissection is needed.

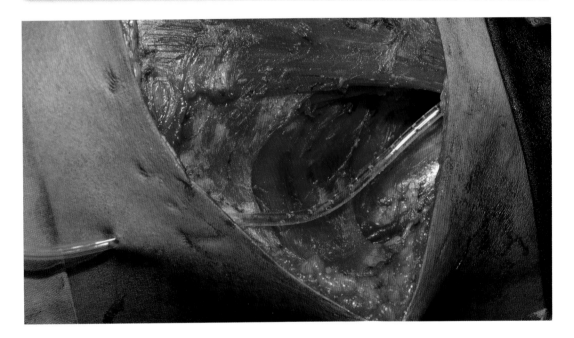

ABOVE Insertion of a drain into the armpit after a mastectomy.

BELOW Surgeons closing the skin after a mastectomy.

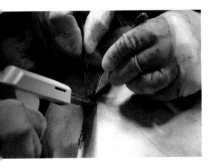

Another reconstruction option is to use part of a back muscle (latissimus dorsi) with a silicone implant. Alternatively, an inflatable tissue expander may be inserted to stretch the skin — this is later replaced with a silicone or saline implant.

While many surgeons are trained to perform mastectomy, reconstructive breast surgery is a highly skilled procedure. It is often performed by a specialist plastic surgeon working together with your breast surgeon.

6 Suction drains are placed in the operation area to prevent a build-up of fluid *(see above)*. The wound is then closed without tension, using stitches or staples *(see left)*, taking care not to leave any unnecessary flaps of skin at the corners of the incision. A pressure dressing may be applied to minimize oozing after surgery.

LUMPECTOMY/MASTECTOMY
QUESTIONS & ANSWERS

What are the benefits?

When detected early, at a localized stage that has not yet spread beyond the breast, the five-year survival rate for breast cancer is 98%, and the ten-year survival rate is 90%. These survival rates are similar for lumpectomy or mastectomy.

What are the risks?

As well as the general risks associated with surgery and general anesthesia *(see pages 10–11)*, you may develop numbness of the skin over the breast area. Occasionally, the tissue may break down so you need another operation to revise the scar. Removal of tissues in the armpit can lead to swelling of the arm with lymph fluid (lymphedema) and may injure nerves that control feeling and movement in parts of the arm and hand. Most women recover with no complications, however.

The chance of a long-term breast cancer recurrence within 20 years is 15% to 20% with lumpectomy and radiation therapy, and is lower at 3% to 5% with mastectomy. It is possible that skin- and nipple-sparing mastectomy, which leave behind more tissue, may slightly increase the long-term risk of breast cancer recurrence, within 20 years, by an additional 1% to 2%. However, newer hormonal therapies, chemotherapy, and biological therapies are continually improving the chances of recurrence-free, long-term survival. An early detection plan that includes self-examination, clinical breast examination, and screening mammography is vital *(see page 84)*. It is important to continue checking both breasts after lumpectomy, and the remaining breast after mastectomy.

Are there any alternatives?

A number of surgical and medical options are available, as described in the preceding pages.

What can I do to prepare?

Try to be as fit and healthy as possible. If you smoke, do your utmost to stop to reduce the risk of complications. Try to maintain a positive frame of mind, and take an active part in discussions with your surgeon to decide the best treatment options for you. If you decide to have a mastectomy, consider whether or not you wish to have an immediate or a delayed breast reconstruction.

What if I don't have the operation?

Your surgeon will advise the likely outcome of not having a lumpectomy or mastectomy, based on the type of cancer cells present and their aggressiveness. Treatment with radiotherapy, chemotherapy, and/or drugs may help to contain the tumor. In most cases, however, the best outcome is obtained by removing the tumor, either by means of lumpectomy or mastectomy, followed by individually tailored medical treatment.

What happens during the recovery period?

You will receive pain relief either orally or through an intravenous drip. The drains are removed once they stop collecting fluid. You can usually go home as soon as you feel ready. Any non-dissolving stitches or clips are removed around seven days after the operation.

You may progress to further medical treatment, such as radiotherapy, anti-estrogen hormone therapy (for example with the drug, tamoxifen), chemotherapy, or biological therapy using a monoclonal antibody. Known as trastuzumab, this antibody is used to treat advanced breast cancer in women whose tumors produce an abnormally high amount of a protein called HER2. For up to 30% of women with breast cancer, trastuzumab helps to slow tumor growth and can prolong survival compared with chemotherapy alone. It will not help if your HER2 levels are normal, however.

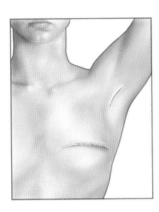

ABOVE A diagram showing the appearance of the human breast after a mastectomy.

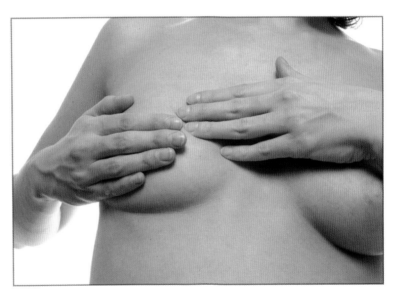

RIGHT Examining your breasts for lumps can help the early detection of breast cancer.

Breast cancer check points

Some breasts are naturally more lumpy than others, and may change at different times of your monthly cycle. By learning how your breasts feel at different times, however, subtle changes can be detected. A good time to be aware of your breasts is when you are in the bath, shower, or when dressing.

Examine your breasts regularly.
• Get to know their normal look and feel.
• Look out for any lumps, dimpling, thickening, or change in shape and size.
• Attend for regular breast screening mammography.
• If you notice any changes, seek medical advice straight away.

You can create your own Early Detection Plan at www.nationalbreastcancer.org

APPENDECTOMY

Appendectomy (or appendicectomy) is the removal of the appendix. The appendix is a blind-ending pouch that branches off from the cecum, which is the first part of the large bowel. The appendix averages 4 in (10 cm) in length, but can vary between 0.8 in and 8.5 in (2 cm and 22 cm). Because of its long, thin shape, it is referred to as the vermiform (worm-like) appendix, or vermix. Although it is often viewed as a vestigial organ left over from ancient times, it contains lymphoid tissue and may play a role in gut immunity. It also acts as a reservoir for healthy digestive bacteria (lactobacilli) to replenish the gut after taking antibiotics, or after a vomiting and diarrhea illness (gastroenteritis). However, people who have their appendix removed do not seem to come to any harm as a result.

WHEN IS APPENDECTOMY NEEDED?

The appendix is taken out when it becomes infected and inflamed. Known as appendicitis, this causes severe abdominal pain. This typically starts with mid-abdominal pain that slowly worsens. Loss of appetite, rapid pulse, and a fever may follow. Cramping sensations can occur and most people (90%) develop nausea and vomiting. A few (10%) also experience diarrhea. The surgeon may smell your breath as this may have a characteristic "fecal" odor. Once inflammation spreads to the surface of the appendix, the pain becomes localized in the lower right-hand side of the abdomen (right iliac fossa). In one in four people, the pain is always felt in the lower right-hand side, rather than shifting there from the belly button area.

Appendectomy may be carried out routinely during other abdominal operations as a preventive measure against the future development of appendicitis. This is less common now that it has been found useful as a "spare part" during some reconstruction operations. The benefits of this procedure — known as incidental appendectomy — decrease significantly in people over the age of 30.

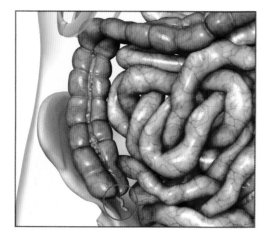

BELOW A diagram showing the position of the appendix (circled in red).

APPENDECTOMY AT A GLANCE

• *Can it be done as an outpatient?* No. Admission to hospital is necessary.

• *Do I need a general anesthetic?* Yes.

• *What special tests are needed?* Diagnosis is based on symptoms and clinical examination. A rectal examination is performed to detect any tenderness and swelling in the appendix area. In women an "internal" or pelvic examination is also needed. Blood tests are performed to look for signs of infection (high white blood cell count) and, in women of fertile age, a pregnancy test is important to exclude ectopic pregnancy. A pelvic ultrasound, CT (computed tomography) scan, and/or diagnostic laparoscopy may be carried out before proceeding to appendectomy if the diagnosis remains uncertain. As the appendix can be removed via laparoscopy *(see page 97)*, some surgeons always use an initial laparoscopic examination in women of fertile age, as one third of young women with symptoms suggestive of appendicitis turn out to have another gynecological cause for their pain.

• *How long does the surgery take?* From 20 minutes to one hour or more, depending on the size and position of the appendix, and degree of inflammation.

• *What is the mortality rate?* Less than one in 100 (0.12%)

• *How long will I be in hospital?* Patients usually stay in hospital for an average of two to three days.

• *How expensive is it?* 💲

• *How many are performed in the US each year?* Around 300,000 operations are performed in the US each year. It is the most common emergency procedure for abdominal pain. Appendicitis is most common between the ages of ten and 30. Before the age of 25, males are twice as likely to develop appendicitis as females; after this age the balance slowly shifts toward equal numbers. Overall, slightly more operations are performed on males (54%). Around one in ten people have their appendix removed at some time during their life.

WHAT CAUSES APPENDICITIS?

Appendicitis develops when the narrow opening along its length (the lumen) becomes blocked. This may result from swelling of lymphoid tissue in the wall of the appendix, or from a build-up of "dried" impacted bowel contents which can cause an obstruction. Blockage encourages bacterial overgrowth within the appendix, leading to infection.

Unusual symptoms

If the appendix is long, it may extend between the intestines, or down into the pelvis. This can cause urinary symptoms if the bladder becomes involved, or may mimic food poisoning with diffuse abdominal pain, vomiting, and diarrhea. Appendicitis can also cause unusual symptoms in young children and in the elderly, who tend to experience pain in a different way. The diagnosis can be confused by other conditions mimicking appendicitis pain, especially gynecological (female) problems, such as a ruptured ovarian cyst, an ectopic pregnancy (a pregnancy developing in a Fallopian tube), or pelvic inflammatory disease (infection of the Fallopian tubes that connect the ovaries to the uterus).

Similarly, appendicitis must always be considered in any pregnant woman who develops abdominal pain, as the enlarged uterus pushes the appendix into the upper abdomen.

In children, inflammation of lymph nodes in the abdomen (mesenteric adenitis) is often misdiagnosed as appendicitis.

Appendectomy
Step-by-step

Open appendectomy

Fluid replacement is needed via a drip as most patients are dehydrated having had little food or drink during the previous 24 hours. Intravenous antibiotics are given at the beginning of the operation — as a single dose for an uncomplicated "early" appendicitis that has not perforated, or as a three to five day course where perforation or gangrene has occurred.

The length of the appendix, and the position of its tip, are variable, but its base is usually found in the same area. Known as McBurney's point, this is located two-thirds of the distance from the belly button (umbilicus) to the tip of the right hip bone (anteriosuperior iliac spine). This is where the incision is usually made. Before making a cut the surgeon will re-examine your abdomen when you are anesthetized and your muscles are relaxed. He may feel a mass that was not detectable before, and may decide to make the incision elsewhere as a result.

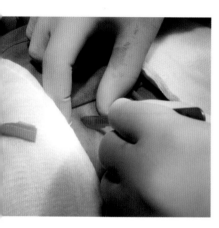

ABOVE **Making the first incision.**

❶ The incision most commonly used for appendectomy is a short cut over the site of McBurney's point. The traditional incision is made diagonally, and is around 2 in to 3 in (5 cm to 8 cm) long. Most surgeons now use a more horizontal cut, however, in a skin crease *(see left)*, as this gives a better cosmetic result, can be extended more easily when wide access is needed, and is associated with a lower rate of wound infection. Occasionally a midline incision is made if the patient is very obese, or if the surgeon suspects that the appendix has ruptured at its base, or that part of the bowel needs to be removed, too.

❷ After cutting the skin, and underlying subcutaneous fat *(see opposite above)*, the three layers of muscle in the abdominal wall (external oblique, internal oblique, and transverse muscles) are split in the direction of their fibers, to avoid cutting the muscles as much as possible. The surgeon opens up the wound and uses his or her fingers to pull the split muscles apart in the direction of their fibers. This is known as a gridiron incision, and exposes the underlying peritoneal membrane which lines the abdominal cavity. Any bleeding points are sealed with heat (diathermy).

Re-assessing the diagnosis

In a small number of patients, no appendix is present — either because it did not develop, or because it has withered away (atrophied). In this case, the surgeon needs to look for other causes of the patient's abdominal symptoms. Similarly, if the appendix looks normal (up to 20% of cases) it is nevertheless removed *(see page 96)* and other diagnoses are carefully sought by inspecting the bowel, pancreas, gallbladder, pelvic organs, and abdominal lymph nodes. If bile is seen in the abdominal cavity, the surgeon looks for a perforated peptic ulcer or gallbladder. The surgeon always remains prepared to close his original incision and make a new one (e.g. for a laparotomy) depending on his or her findings.

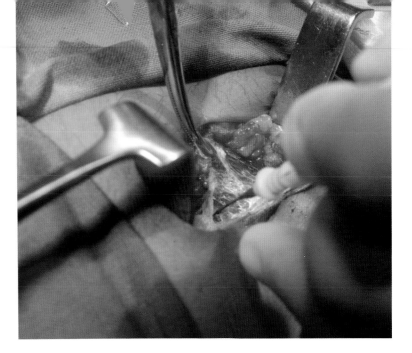

RIGHT Cutting through the subcutaneous fat.

3 An assistant holds the edges of the wound firmly open with a retractor, and the surgeon carefully picks up a fold of peritoneal membrane with toothed forceps. After ensuring no bowel is attached, he makes an incision in the membrane to enter the abdominal cavity *(see below)*. Any visible pus is swabbed and sent to the laboratory for microscopy and culture. This helps to identify the organism involved and the antibiotics to which they are sensitive. The edges of the wound are protected with moistened swabs, and the surgeon looks for the cecum, which forms the pouch-like beginning of the large bowel. From here, the surgeon follows a longitudinal band of muscle (anterior taenia) on the front of the cecum down to the base of the appendix.

BELOW An assistant surgeon holds the wound open with retractors as the surgeon identifies the appendix.

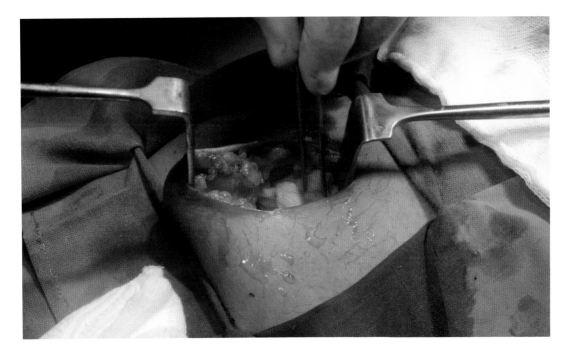

4 The appendix is gently lifted and delivered through the wound to rest on the patient's abdomen, taking care not to rupture it as any adhesions are carefully pulled away *(see left)*. It is always coaxed out by pushing from within, not pulling from without, as pulling on a gangrenous appendix can cause it to rupture. If it is not easily accessible, the surgeon may have to extend his incision. If rupture does occur, the surgeon carefully washes out any escaped material and may insert a drain to encourage healing. This will be removed post-operatively once it has stopped draining any fluid.

5 The appendix is grasped carefully with tissue forceps and held against the light to identify the artery that supplies it with blood. This lies in a small fan of tissues (mesoappendix) that run between the length of the appendix and the cecum. This fan of tissue is clamped, tied, and cut. The base of the appendix is then crushed, clamped, and tied off before the appendix is

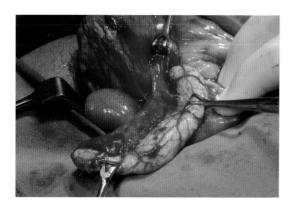

ABOVE Pulling out the appendix.

BELOW Cutting out the appendix.

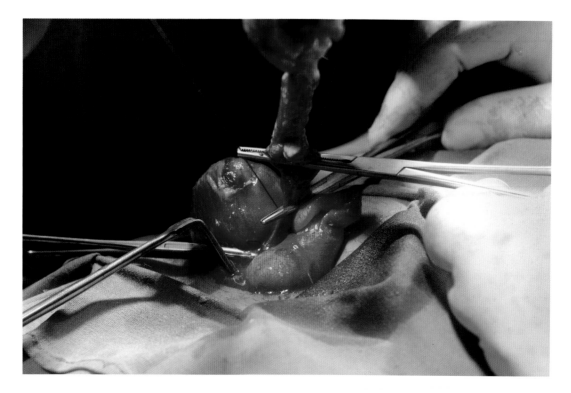

Normal appendix

If a normal appendix is found during a classic appendectomy operation, it is almost always removed, unless bowel inflammation is present (e.g. Crohn's disease). Otherwise, if the patient develops appendicitis in the future, the diagnosis is likely to be discounted if a classic appendectomy scar is present. Doctors will assume the appendix has already been removed.

Laparoscopic appendectomy

The appendix is now usually removed laparoscopically using a viewing device called a laparoscope. This is performed when the diagnosis is uncertain or when a patient has a lot of abdominal fat which would mean having to make a large incision if the appendix was removed by means of the traditional route. Some evidence suggests post-operative hospital stays may be slightly shorter using this approach, as many people having a routine appendectomy can go home the day after the operation. This is also true of the traditional approach, however, assuming the patient is well-hydrated and the appendix, when revealed, was "normal" or only mildly inflamed. Where the patient is "toxic" and showing signs of infection with symptoms including fever and a rapid pulse, they will need to stay in hospital until the infection is under control.

cut away *(see opposite below)*. A special purse-string stitch is then sewn circularly into the cecum, around the remaining stump of the appendix. This is pulled tight as the stump is pushed inside to safely enclose the stump (which may be inflamed) within a wall of healthy tissue. If it is considered unsafe to insert a purse-string in the cecum (for example, if it is also inflamed), a piece of omentum (fatty tissue hanging down from the intestines) may be sewn over the stump instead.

❻ Once the appendix is safely removed, and all bleeding has been stopped, the edges of the peritoneum are closed with a continuous stitch. The wound is then cleansed with an antiseptic. Loose, interrupted (separate) stitches are then used to close the inner two layers of abdominal muscle. The outer layer of muscle/tendon is sewn with a loose continuous stitch and the skin closed with a concealed running stitch beneath the skin (subcuticular suture) or clips *(see below)*.

RIGHT Closing the wound.

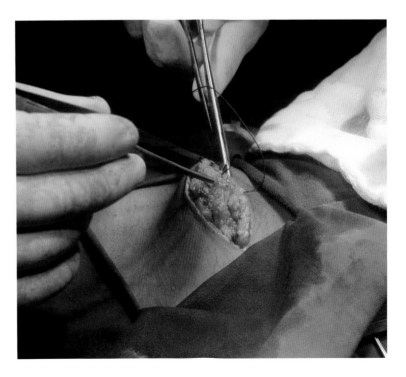

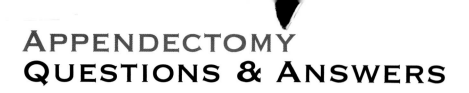

APPENDECTOMY
QUESTIONS & ANSWERS

What are the benefits?

Appendectomy is usually a life-saving operation. When performed early, it prevents perforation of the appendix and significantly reduces the risk of developing an abscess and septicemia (blood poisoning).

What are the risks?

As well as the general risks associated with surgery and general anesthesia *(see pages 10–11)*, there is a risk of bowel perforation during surgery. If the appendix is gangrenous, there is an increased risk of wound infection. Rarely, an opening (fistula) may form between the stump of the appendix and the abdominal wall, which leaks feces. This is treated by inserting a large tube to protect the edges of the opening. After a week, when inflammation has settled down, the tube is removed and the fistula usually heals spontaneously.

Are there any alternatives?

Not really, if the diagnosis is certain, the inflamed appendix needs to be removed. If the diagnosis is uncertain, despite computed tomography (CT) scanning of the abdomen, a laparoscopy or laparotomy may be performed.

What can I do to prepare?

If you have increasing abdominal pain and may need an operation, you are usually advised to remain "nil by mouth." By not eating or drinking, your stomach is empty making a general anesthetic safer if you need an urgent operation for suspected appendicitis.

What if I don't have the operation?

If not treated, infection can lead to gangrene and perforation of the appendix. This can lead to widespread infection of the abdomen (peritonitis) and blood poisoning (septicemia) which is life-threatening. Sometimes, an appendix mass forms when the inflamed appendix becomes "walled off" by the omentum (a fatty sheet of tissue hanging down from the intestines). When this is diagnosed, the outline of the mass is marked out on the abdomen and closely monitored to ensure it does not get progressively bigger. If the patient is relatively well, with no signs of septicemia, treatment is conservative, with antibiotics injected straight into a vein. If an ultrasound or computed tomography

Latest technique

Surgeons in San Diego are developing a technique called "natural orifice transluminal surgery" or NOTES, in which an appendix, or other diseased internal organs, can be removed by an incision made through the body's natural openings, such as the mouth and stomach, vagina, or rectum.

If, for any reason, your appendix was not removed (for example, if the surgeon found your symptoms were due to Crohn's disease — an inflammatory disease of the bowel), you will be warned to inform any future doctors that your appendix is still present (despite you having a typical appendectomy scar).

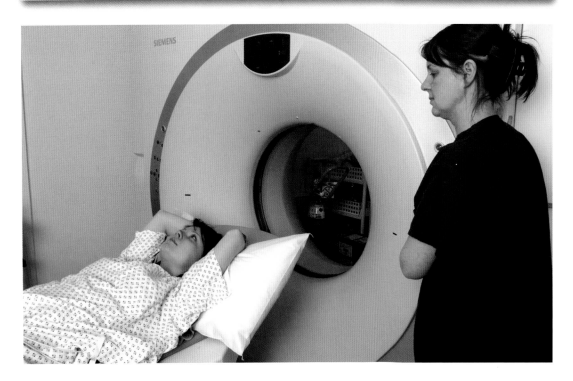

ABOVE A female patient is prepared for a CT scan.

(CT) scan shows that an abscess has formed, this may be drained via a needle inserted through the skin (or rectum) under ultrasound control. If the patient's condition worsens, an open operation may be needed to drain the abscess. Once symptoms have settled, the appendix may be removed at a later date, one to two months later. Increasingly, however, interval appendectomy is only carried out if symptoms start to flare up again, which is relatively rare. This is because there is often no evidence of the appendix when an interval operation is carried out — the body has "digested" it and the remains have withered away (atrophied).

What happens during the recovery period?

As long as there is no widespread infection (peritonitis), you can start drinking fluids and eating a light diet as soon as you are fully awake and feel ready. If peritonitis is present, you will be kept "nil by mouth" and receive fluids and antibiotics through a drip straight into your veins, until the infection settles. If the appendix was perforated, you will receive a course of antibiotics, typically for five days. If a drain was in place, it is removed after two to three days (or later, if it is still draining).

You can usually return to work within seven to ten days, but sometimes it may take three weeks or longer if you had suffered from widespread infection.

COLORECTAL RESECTION

The surgical removal, or resection, of part of the large bowel may be needed to treat cancer of the colon or rectum, or the complications of inflammatory conditions such as Crohn's disease, ulcerative colitis, and severe diverticulitis. Occasionally, it is needed to remove an air-filled segment of the bowel that has become twisted (volvulus) and died due to lack of blood supply, or a rectal prolapse in which part of the rectum slips out through the anus.

THE LARGE INTESTINES

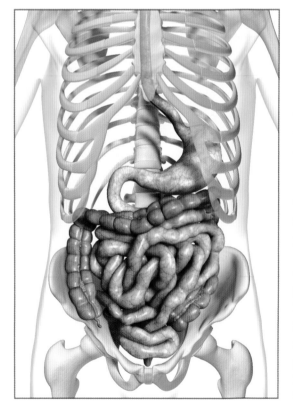

BELOW A diagram showing the position of the colon below the stomach in the abdominal cavity.

The colon and rectum form the large intestines, also known as the hind gut or large bowel. It is made up of five main parts, starting with the pouch-like cecum. This leads into the ascending colon (which passes up the right side of the abdomen), the transverse colon (which crosses the top of the abdominal cavity), and on to the descending colon (which passes down the left side of the abdominal cavity). The final part forms a curve, the sigmoid colon, which leads into the rectum.

Bowel contents arriving in the cecum from the small intestines form a semi-liquid slurry from which most nutrients have been absorbed. The large intestines extract excess fluid, salts, and minerals and, at the same time, bacteria present within the colon ferment undigested fiber to break it down. Of around 4 pints (2 liters) of bowel contents received into the colon each day, only around 0.5 pint (250 ml) of semi-solid waste remains. When this enters the last part of the large bowel, the rectum, it triggers a voiding reflex that takes you to the bathroom.

Cancer of the colon or rectum is the most common reason for needing a colorectal resection. An estimated 145,000 new cases of bowel cancer are diagnosed in the United States each year, of which around 105,000 are in the colon, and 40,000 in the rectum. The good news is that routine screening of the population means this condition is often picked up at an early, potentially curable stage.

COLORECTAL RESECTION AT A GLANCE

- **Can it be done as an outpatient?** No. Admission to hospital is necessary.

- **Do I need a general anesthetic?** Yes.

- **What special tests are needed?** Every attempt is made to obtain a biopsy sample of diseased areas of bowel to confirm the suspected diagnosis, using a viewing device inserted through the anus. Sigmoidoscopy can examine the sigmoid colon, descending colon, and rectum; colonoscopy can examine the entire length of the colon. Virtual colonoscopy, in which X-rays and computers are used to generate a view of the colon and rectum, may be available as an alternative to help plan the surgery.
  - For rectal tumors, ultrasound using a rectal probe (transrectal ultrasonography) helps to determine whether the tumor has spread through the rectal wall. Examination of the bladder (cystoscopy) may also be needed to see if it is involved.
  - Chest X-ray and abdominal/pelvic computed tomography (CT) scanning or positron emission tomography (PET) is performed to look for distant spread (metastasis) of the disease.

- A blood test to measure a substance called carcinoembryonic antigen (CEA) is performed as part of the staging evaluation for bowel cancer. Levels of CEA should return to normal after surgical resection; if they rise again during follow-up, this suggests a recurrence of the tumor.

- **How long does the surgery take?** Conventional abdominal surgery takes from one to three hours, depending on the procedure, and what is found during the operation. A laparoscopic procedure usually takes around 40 minutes longer than the traditional approach.

- **What is the mortality rate?** Around one in 25 (4%).

- **How long will I be in hospital?** Patients usually stay in hospital for an average of ten days.

- **How expensive is it?** $ $ $

- **How many are performed in the US each year?** Around 285,000 operations are performed in the US each year. It is most common in men and women over the age of 45. Just over half the operations are in female patients.

SCREENING FOR BOWEL CANCER

Screening for bowel cancer can involve a digital rectal examination, in which a doctor inserts a finger to detect any ulcer or mass in the rectum; fecal occult blood tests (which look for signs of hidden blood in the feces); dual-contrast barium enema (an imaging technique which uses X-rays to outline the bowel wall), and sigmoidoscopy or total colonoscopy in which a viewing device is inserted through the anus to view the bowel directly (biopsies can also be taken with this technique). Routine screening using fecal occult blood testing is usually recommended annually from the age of 50 years. Sigmoidoscopy may be suggested every five years, and screening colonoscopy every ten years. High risk individuals may need more frequent screening.

Symptoms

Symptoms of bowel cancer vary, but can include:
- Change in bowel habit, such as change in frequency, constipation or diarrhea.
- Blood and/or mucus in the stools.
- Anemia and fatigue.
- Bloating.
- Cramping bowel pains or discomfort.
- Weight loss.
- Many early bowel cancers do not cause symptoms, however, and are found during routine screening or surveillance.

COLORECTAL RESECTION
STEP-BY-STEP

PARTIAL OR TOTAL COLECTOMY

Bowel preparation is usually carried out before surgery to reduce the number of bacteria (e.g. *Escherichia coli, Bacteroides fragilis*) within the colon. Emptying the bowel also makes it easier to manipulate during surgery. Powerful laxatives are given along with large volumes of clear liquids, typically at noon and 6 pm on the day before the operation. A more gentle bowel preparation, designed for people with heart, liver, or kidney problems, may be given early on the day before surgery. Alternatively, an enema may be used to clear the lower bowel of any accumulation of hard stools.

A hemicolectomy is where half the colon is removed. Depending on the disease and its position, a surgeon may perform a left hemicolectomy (upper part of the descending colon and left half of the transverse colon) or a right hemicolectomy (cecum, ascending colon, and right half of the transverse colon). Other procedures that are possible include resection of the entire transverse colon (transverse colectomy, or as part of an extended left or right hemicolectomy), resection of the sigmoid colon (sigmoid colectomy), or removal of the whole colon (total colectomy). The upper rectum is removed in a procedure called an anterior resection.

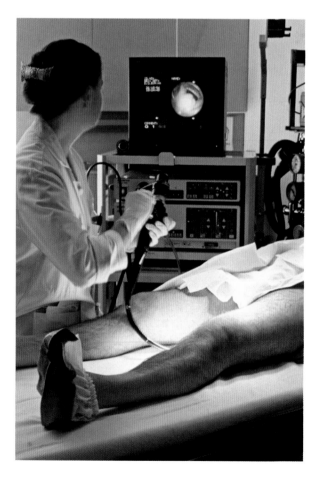

BELOW A doctor examines an image of a patient's colon obtained using a fiber-optic viewing device (colonoscope).

Where possible, the surgeon will try to join up (anastomose) the cut ends on either side of the resected bowel. If this is not possible, for example because of poor blood supply, too much tension, or because the lower end of the rectum is involved, the surgeon may fashion a colostomy which can be temporary, or permanent *(see page 104).* The surgeon may mark possible sites for a colostomy opening (stoma) on the front wall of the abdomen at the start of the operation (avoiding belt lines, scars etc) even if the need for one is not anticipated.

Intravenous antibiotics are given at the time of anesthesia to reduce risk of infection after cutting the bowel. A blood thinning agent is also given to reduce the risk of deep vein thrombosis. A catheter is inserted into the bladder to keep it empty during the operation.

❶ The abdomen is opened through a midline incision that extends from 0.8 in (2 cm) below the ribs to 2 in (5 cm) above the pubic bone, swerving around the belly button to the right. After controlling any bleeding points, the surgeon may clip moist wound towels to the skin edges to protect them from contamination. He or she then cuts down through the abdominal layers using a knife or hot (diathermy) blade. Finally, the peritoneal membrane lining the abdominal cavity is carefully picked up with toothed forceps. After ensuring no bowel is attached, it is cut open to enter the abdominal cavity. Any visible pus is swabbed and sent to the laboratory for microscopy and culture. This helps to identify the organism involved and the antibiotics to which they are sensitive. The surgeon then thoroughly explores the internal organs, especially the liver (a common site for metastatic spread of a bowel cancer).

❷ The segment of bowel to be removed is mobilized, and its main blood vessels are tied and cut. The length of bowel that is to be cut away (resected) is clamped or stapled closed. The ends of the bowel that will remain inside are closed with non-crushing clamps (to help avoid contamination with bowel contents) and the ends are cleaned with antiseptic swabs.

BELOW Surgeons remove cancerous tissue from the lining of the colon (local resection).

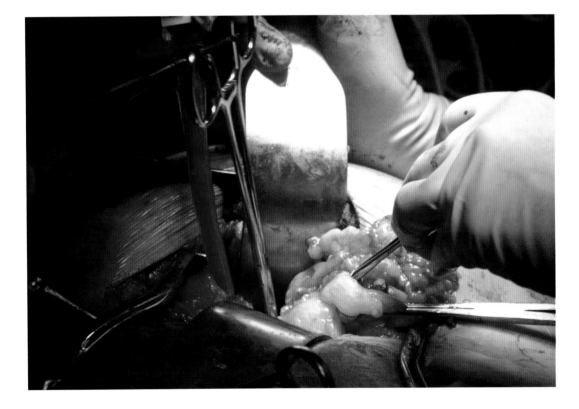

Abdominoperineal excision

If a rectal cancer is situated low down, near the anus, it may be removed using a double approach. One surgical team operates on the abdomen to fashion a colostomy, while the other team operates through the perineum to remove the rectum and anus. In a female, the back wall of the vagina is usually removed, too. This is known as an abdominoperineal excision.

ASSESSING THE EXTENT OF RESECTION

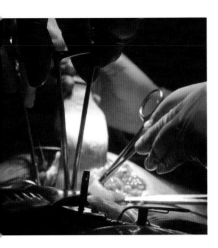

❸ The diseased area of colon/rectum and any structures stuck to it are cut away *(see left)*. This may sometimes include a loop of small bowel, an ovary, uterus, or kidney if they have been invaded by cancerous tissue. If curative resection is not possible, palliative resection is carried out to remove as much diseased tissue as possible. If this is not feasible, then a bypass is performed to re-route bowel contents around any areas of disease and narrowing.

❹ The remaining bowel ends are trimmed to a similar size and either sewn together or stapled, ensuring there is no twist in the bowel and that the ends are not under tension. After completion of this step, swabs, towels, gloves, and instruments are changed to reduce risk of contamination. A drain is usually left in place to help prevent a build-up of infected fluid that may lead to the formation of an abscess.

ABOVE Surgeons performing bowel surgery on a patient with colon cancer.

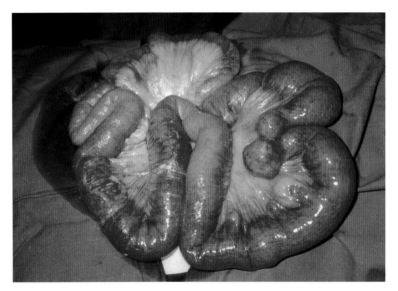

RIGHT Bowel cancer may cause an obstruction causing the intestines to become dilated.

Colostomy and ileostomy

- A colostomy connects part of the large bowel (colon) to an opening (stoma) made in the abdominal wall, usually on the left-hand side. Waste is semi-solid or solid and collected in a colostomy pouch which sticks to the abdominal wall. This is replaced one to three times a day.
- An ileostomy connects the end of the small bowel (ileum) to an opening made in the abdominal wall, usually on the right-hand side, to form a "spout." Waste is soft or liquid, and collected in a pouch that can be drained from a sealable opening at regular intervals.

- A temporary colostomy or ileostomy may be needed to give damaged or operated bowel time to rest and heal. It is closed by a subsequent operation several weeks later, after all swelling has settled down.
- A permanent colostomy may be needed if a cancer cannot be completely removed, if the two ends of bowel cannot be sewn together, or if the lower rectum is involved.
- A permanent ileostomy is needed following a total colectomy.

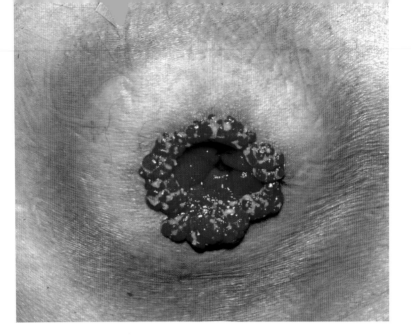

RIGHT A healed wound and colostomy opening (stoma).

5 If a colostomy is needed, this is fashioned by making an opening in the abdominal wall, through which a loop of bowel is pulled. The loop is slit open and the edges turned back and sewn to the abdominal wall. This leaves a red, moist opening that has no feeling *(see above)*. A temporary "loop" ileostomy is made in a similar way. A permanent ileostomy is made by pulling the end of the small bowel (ileum) through a small hole made in the abdominal wall. It is sewn into place to form a small spout which projects around 1.2 in (3 cm) from the abdominal wall.

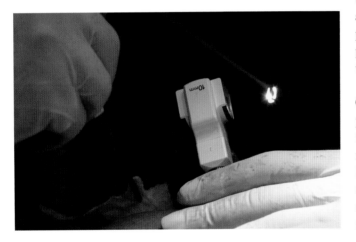

BELOW A surgeon prepares to insert a laparoscope through an incision in the abdominal wall.

6 After checking no other procedures are needed, the incision is closed using the surgeon's referred method, either layer by layer, or as one simple mass closure except for the skin. The skin is then closed with stitches or staples, and the wound is dressed.

Laparoscopic colorectal resection

Increasing numbers of people are now having a laparoscopic resection. Four or more small punctures are made in the abdominal wall, and the surgeon inserts and manipulates special instruments guided via a video-endoscope (viewing device) *(see above)*. Benefits include less pain, more rapid return to normal bowel function, less tiredness, and improved convalescence. Research shows that laparoscopic resection has similar results to open resection for time to tumor recurrence, wound involvement, and overall survival at four and a half years. Laparoscopic surgery takes an average of 40 minutes longer than the conventional approach.

COLORECTAL RESECTION
QUESTIONS & ANSWERS

What are the benefits?

The operation removes diseased bowel. This gives you the best chance of a cure for some diseases, such as bowel cancer. It can also significantly improve bowel symptoms, such as pain.

What are the risks?

As well as the general risks associated with surgery and general anesthesia *(see pages 10–11)*, handling the small bowel can lead to paralytic ileus, in which it is slow to start working again after surgery. This is treated by maintaining fluids only to "rest" the bowel. A nasogastric tube may be passed to prevent vomiting. There is a risk of anastomotic leak at the site where the bowel was rejoined. This is treated with antibiotics and bowel "rest." Sometimes surgery is needed to form a temporary colostomy until the leak heals. Surgery for rectal cancer can lead to impotence in males, due to nerve damage. This can be treated with a prosthesis (penile implant) one year after surgery if the pelvis is free from recurrence.

RIGHT **This patient has undergone a colectomy and colostomy for perforated diverticulitis. A drain is siphoning pus from a pelvic abscess that developed after surgery.**

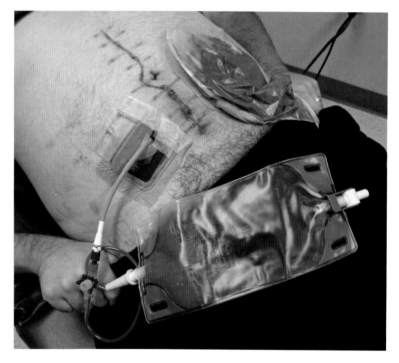

Are there any alternatives?

Radiotherapy or chemotherapy may be suggested to treat bowel cancer, but these usually work better if the cancer is also removed surgically. Radiotherapy before rectal surgery can improve survival and decrease recurrences. Rectal tumors can sometimes be treated with excision, heat, radiation, and laser vaporization through the anus.

What can I do to prepare?

Try to be as fit and healthy as possible. Eat a well-balanced diet, unless advised to follow a particular eating regime by your physicians. Take gentle exercise. If you smoke, do your utmost to stop.

What if I don't have the operation?

If surgery is not carried out when recommended by your surgeon, it is likely that you will experience a worsening of your symptoms, and of your health. Depending on the bowel disease you have, you may develop a blockage, a perforated bowel, or an abscess, all of which are potentially life-threatening. If you have cancer, it is more likely to spread and become incurable.

What happens during the recovery period?

After surgery you will have a number of tubes coming from your body, which may include an intravenous infusion (drip), bladder catheter, drainage tubes at the site of operation, a nasogastric tube through the nose to the stomach, and an oxygen source. You may have a pump that releases pain relief (patient controlled analgesia) when you need it. Most of these tubes are removed over the next one to five days. You can start eating and drinking as soon as your bowel function returns to normal, which may take a few days. Visible stitches or clips are removed after seven to 12 days.

You are likely to feel tired during the first few weeks after surgery, but gentle mobilization is important to reduce the risk of deep vein blood clots. You will be advised not to lift anything heavy, or to carry out strenuous activities, for at least the first six weeks. You should not drive until you are advised that you can do so by your doctor and insurance provider. This is usually once you can perform an emergency stop without fear that your wound may hurt.

You may experience urgency, constipation, diarrhea, or loose stools after surgery, which usually settles down. Medication can help to control these bowel symptoms.

When, or if, you can return to work depends on the bowel condition that you have, and the type of work that you do.

Chemotherapy

Chemotherapy is a standard post-operative treatment for advanced cancers which involve lymph nodes (Stage III) or which have spread more distantly (Stage IV).

Regular follow-up is needed after surgery to detect any recurrences. This usually involves surveillance colonoscopy the first year after resection, then every three years, then every five years if remaining negative. Blood levels of carcinoembryonic antigen (CEA) are usually checked and, if they rise, a CT scan, chest X-ray, and positron emmission tomography (PET) scan are needed to identify any recurrence.

Coronary Artery Bypass Graft

Coronary artery disease (CAD) reduces the blood supply to the heart so that heart muscle does not get all the oxygen and nutrients it needs. This results in the symptoms of angina. If the blood supply is totally blocked, a heart attack occurs in which some heart muscle cells will die.

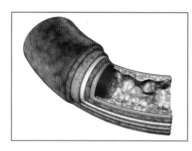

ABOVE **Cross-section through an artery showing the build up of plaque.**

A coronary artery bypass graft — also known as a CABG or simply a bypass — provides a new blood supply to the affected parts of the heart before long-term damage occurs. A new blood vessel (the graft) is attached to run from the body's main artery, the aorta, to a point in the coronary artery beyond the area of narrowing. This allows blood to flow around, or bypass, the blockage. The graft is usually made from a healthy, non-essential blood vessel taken from the chest wall (internal thoracic artery), leg (great saphenous vein), or arm (radial artery). Depending on whether one, two, three, four, or five coronary arteries are bypassed, it is known as a single, double, triple, quadruple, or quintuple bypass operation.

What causes coronary artery disease?

Hardening and narrowing of the coronary arteries (atherosclerosis) results when a sticky build-up of porridge-like cholesterol and calcium (atheroma) forms on the inner walls of the arteries. This reduces the blood flow to heart muscle cells. In some people, two-thirds or more of a coronary artery may be blocked with atheroma without causing symptoms. Others may experience angina even though only a small amount of plaque is present and their coronary artery is only narrowed slightly. It all depends on:

• The exact site of the narrowing.
• Whether one or more coronary arteries are affected.
• How well your coronary arteries join up to share the load of supplying blood.
• The type of coronary arteries you have inherited — whether they are the vascular equivalent of freeways, or winding country backroads.

Symptoms of angina

Angina feels like a tight pressure, heaviness, or dull ache behind the breastbone. Discomfort may spread through the chest, into the neck, jaw, or down the left arm. It is typically brought on by exertion or strong emotions, and usually fades within a few minutes of resting. Heart attack pain is similar to angina but:

• Lasts longer.
• Is more intense.
• Is usually accompanied by sweating, paleness, and breathlessness.
• Can come on at any time and is unrelieved by rest.

CABG AT A GLANCE

- *Can it be done as an outpatient?* No. Admission to hospital is necessary.

- *Do I need a general anesthetic?* Yes.

- *What special tests are needed?* The location of the blockage(s) within the coronary arteries is identified before planning the operation by coronary catheterization and angiography *(see below)*. A narrow tube (catheter) is inserted into an artery in the groin under local anesthetic, while you lie flat on an X-ray table. The catheter is advanced through the circulation, without blocking blood flow, until its tip reaches the opening of the coronary arteries. An X-ray dye is then injected while X-ray images are taken, to outline the coronary arteries and pinpoint the sites of narrowing. This helps the cardiologist to plan the CABG operation. Newer non-invasive methods, such as high speed CT scanning angiography, to visualize the heart arteries are under evaluation.

- *How long does the surgery take?* Three to six hours depending on how many bypass grafts are inserted.

- *What is the mortality rate?* Overall mortality is 3% to 4%. The risk of complications increases in those who are over 70 years of age, have poor heart muscle function, diabetes, lung or kidney disease, and whose left main coronary artery is affected. Women are also considered higher risk as they are usually older at the time of needing CABG surgery, and tend to have narrower coronary arteries.

- *How long will I be in hospital?* The average stay in hospital is nine days.

- *How expensive is it?* 💲💲💲💲💲

- *How many are performed in the US each year?* Around 250,000 CABG procedures are carried out each year. It is one of the most common procedures performed after the age of 65 years. Around 70% of CABG operations are performed on males.

WHO IS AFFECTED?

The risk of developing CAD increases with age, especially in men over 45 and women after the menopause. It progresses most quickly in people who smoke cigarettes, eat a high-fat diet, are overweight, or take little exercise. The risk is also increased if you have high blood pressure, a raised cholesterol level, poorly controlled diabetes, or a family history of CAD.

WHEN IS A CABG NECESSARY?

A CABG is indicated if you have worsening angina, despite drug treatment, multiple areas of coronary artery narrowing, poor heart pumping action as a result of CAD, or narrowing of the left main coronary artery, or its main branch (left anterior descending).

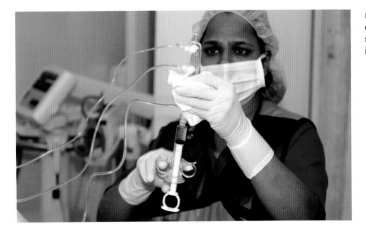

LEFT A member of the coronary catheterization team prepares a control syringe and three-way manifold for use in carrying out an angiography.

CABG
STEP-BY-STEP

GAINING ACCESS TO THE HEART

❶ The surgeon makes an incision down the center of the chest to expose the breastbone, or sternum *(see below)*. The wound is typically around 10 in (25 cm) long. The breastbone is then cut down the middle with a special saw (median sternotomy) and held open with retractors designed to spread the rib cage apart. The surgeon then cuts through the tissues covering the heart, such as the pericardial sac, to expose the beating heart muscle. The surgeon visually inspects the heart before making a final decision about how many arteries to bypass: one, two, three, four, or, occasionally, more.

❷ If the internal thoracic artery is healthy, and free from narrowing, it is selected for use as the graft. It has the advantage of already running from a branch of the aorta close by, so the surgeon just needs to carefully detach its other end from the chest wall for reattachment to the heart. Grafts made from an artery usually perform better, and last longer, than a graft made from a vein. However, sometimes the saphenous leg vein must be used — either because the available arteries are already affected by atherosclerosis, or because multiple grafts are needed. The saphenous vein has the advantage of length and can provide many grafts. However, veins differ from arteries in that they contain internal valves to help prevent the backflow of blood.

RIGHT **A cardiac surgeon incises the skin over the sternum.**

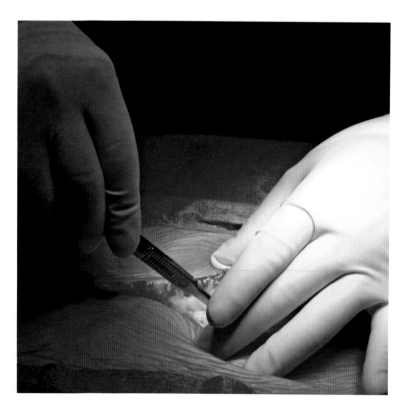

The saphenous vein must therefore have its valves stripped out, or be reversed, so the valves do not obstruct blood flow, if it is to be used as a graft. The lead surgeon will remove and prepare the graft vessel before operating on the heart *(see below)*. Sometimes, one surgeon works on the chest to prepare the heart, while a second surgeon harvests the graft, in order to shorten the operation.

CARDIOPULMONARY BYPASS

❸ Once the graft is ready, the patient's blood is thinned with heparin — a drug that stops unwanted blood clotting. The circulation is then diverted away from the heart to a heart-lung (cardiopulmonary) bypass machine *(see page 112)*, using tubes called cannulae. These are carefully stitched into the large veins (vena cavae) or right atrium of the heart to divert blood to the bypass machine. The bypass machine cools and filters the blood, adds oxygen, and removes waste carbon dioxide before pumping the blood back into the patient's circulation, beyond the heart. Blood flow to the heart itself is stopped by a clamp placed across the aorta. This allows the surgeon to operate on a

BELOW A surgical assistant harvests a patient's greater saphenous vein from the left leg to use as a coronary artery bypass graft.

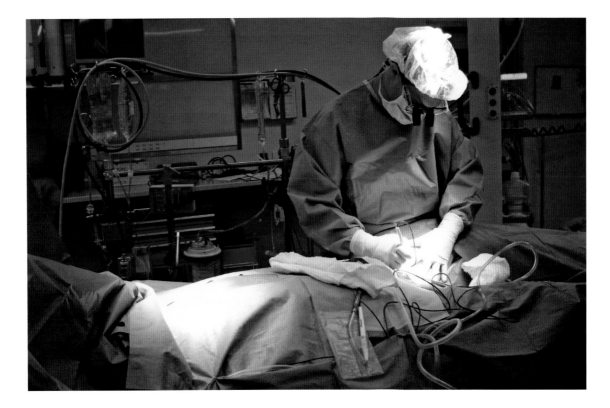

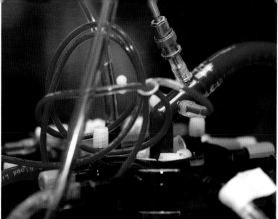

bloodless heart while maintaining circulation to the other vital organs. Cooling the blood down to 93.2 °F (34 °C) (mild hypothermia) is an important step, as it slows the body's metabolism, and reduces the patient's oxygen requirements. A specially trained health professional, called a perfusionist, monitors the bypass machine throughout the operation so the anesthesiologist and surgeons can concentrate on other aspects of the operation.

ABOVE A heart-lung bypass machine routes the patient's blood away from the heart and takes over the heart's pumping action. Surgeons can operate in a relatively blood-free zone, while the patient's organs continue to receive oxygenated blood.

❹ Next, the heart is stopped — a procedure known as cardioplegia — by infusing it with an iced solution (39.2 °F / 4 °C) containing a variety of drugs. This cools the heart and preserves the heart muscle during the operation while its blood supply is severely reduced. The surgeon can now work with a blood-free, immobile heart, making the delicate process of attaching the graft vessel(s) to the heart much easier.

ATTACHING THE GRAFT

❺ The surgeon makes a small incision and carefully stitches one end of the graft to the aorta (unless one of the internal thoracic arteries is used, which is already connected to the aorta). The other end of the graft is stitched to the coronary artery beyond the site of narrowing *(see below)*. Once all the grafts are completed, and the surgeon is happy with the new connections, the clamp is removed from the aorta and blood is allowed to flow back into the heart again. Blood now flows through the grafted coronary artery, bypassing the narrowed area.

RIGHT Surgeons carefully open and inspect one end of the graft, before preparing to stitch it to a coronary artery beyond the site of narrowing.

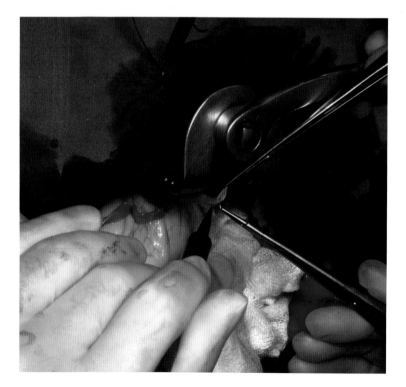

6 The heart is then allowed to start pumping again *(see below)*, either by warming it or by applying a controlled electric shock. Once the heart is beating properly, the heart-lung machine is disconnected and a drug given to reverse the blood-thinning effects of the heparin. The sternum is moved back into place, and the two halves wired together. The surgeon then stitches up the chest wound, usually with dissolvable stitches, or with staple clips which are later removed.

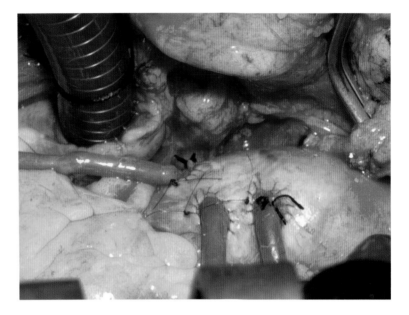

RIGHT The grafts are completed and the heart is allowed to start pumping again. Three coronary artery grafts can be seen, stitched into place, in the bottom half of the picture (a triple bypass).

The number of coronary arteries that are bypassed — one, two, three *(see above)* four or five — depend partly on the degree and position of narrowed areas, and partly on the quality of the coronary arteries. It also depends on their size (those that are less than 0.06 in / 1.5 mm are more difficult to treat), whether or not they are heavily calcified, and whether or not they run within the heart muscle rather than on the heart's surface. These factors can mean that, although a surgeon may have planned to carry out a triple bypass, for example, he actually performs a double or quadruple bypass once he assesses the heart directly.

"Off-pump" bypass surgery

Sometimes, instead of stopping the heart altogether and using a heart-lung bypass machine, the heart is allowed to continue beating but is slowed right down with drugs. This is known as an "off-pump" coronary artery bypass graft or OPCABG. A smaller incision is made in the sternum, and the heart is pulled forward using slings, deep stitches, and special instruments to allow easier access. Bleeding is reduced in the area of operation using sponges, and heart muscle is immobilized near the affected blood vessel using a special suction device that pulls the heart tissue tight. Not using a heart-lung bypass machine appears to reduce the need for blood transfusion and the risk of some complications, such as memory loss and kidney damage, so that the hospital stay is shorter. The procedure is technically more difficult, however, and is not yet routinely available.

CABG
QUESTIONS & ANSWERS

What are the benefits?

In nine out of ten cases, the procedure immediately reduces angina. Many people find that they no longer need angina medications, even during exercise. Having a CABG may also lower the future risk of a heart attack. A successful graft usually lasts between ten and 15 years before re-operation is necessary. Studies suggest that, ten years after CABG surgery, 66% of grafts made from veins are still open, compared with 90% of those made from the internal thoracic arteries.

What are the risks?

As well as the general risks associated with surgery and general anesthesia *(see pages 10–11)*, 5% to 10% of people having a CABG experience a heart attack and 1% to 2% of people experience a stroke. One in four people experience temporary heart rhythm abnormalities within the first three or four days after surgery as a result of trauma to the heart. Kidney problems can also occur. Many people experience temporary depression, poor memory, and difficulty concentrating for a few months, but this usually improves within six months.

Are there any alternatives?

If there is only one area of coronary artery narrowing, you may be offered a percutaneous coronary intervention (PCI — also known as a coronary angioplasty). This involves passing a narrow, balloon-tipped tube into the circulation, and threading it through to the area of narrowing. The balloon is then inflated to widen the artery. At the same time, a small piece of wire-mesh tubing, called a stent, is placed within the artery to keep it open. However, CABG is the preferred treatment where narrowing involves the left main coronary artery, if all three main coronary arteries are affected, if there is diffuse narrowing, and for high risk patients, including those with diabetes.

What can I do to prepare?

Lifestyle modifications are important to help stop CAD progressing *(see below)*. Patients who continue to smoke have a higher risk of wound infection, a slower recovery, and are more likely to need early

Lifestyle modifications

- If you smoke, do your utmost to stop.
- Try to lose some excess weight.
- Try to exercise regularly (e.g. walking) within the limits of your angina — your physician will advise how much exercise you should take.
- Follow a heart-healthy diet supplying plenty of fruit and vegetables — your physician will advise what dietary changes you should make.

repeat surgery. If you have high blood pressure, a raised cholesterol level, or diabetes, it is important that these risk factors for CAD are well controlled with medications.

What if I don't have the operation?

Angina can be controlled with drugs, but CAD is likely to progress and the angina may get worse without surgery.

What happens during the recovery period?

Most patients stay in the intensive care unit for around 24 hours for careful monitoring. Once you return to the ward, you are encouraged to get out of bed and move around to reduce the risk of chest infection and blood clots in the deep veins of the legs. Provided there are no complications, most patients leave hospital within seven to nine days. Some leave within just a few days. You will be advised not to lift heavy objects, and to take care with certain movements, such as pushing yourself out of a chair or reaching up, to avoid stressing the chest wound. Around four to six weeks post-op you will have an exercise stress test in which your heart tracing is monitored while you walk on a treadmill. This will show whether or not your heart muscle is receiving enough oxygen during exercise. If all is well, you can start driving again, and enter a program of cardiac rehabilitation with gradually increasing exercise. You will also receive information on the diet and lifestyle modifications that will help to keep your graft working for as long as possible. Regular follow-up angiography tests will monitor how well the graft is working. Treatment with low-dose aspirin (to thin the blood) and a statin drug (to lower cholesterol levels) is usually recommended.

BELOW Angioplasty is the mechanical widening of a narrowed or totally obstructed blood vessel. The balloon catheter is moved into or near the blockage. The balloon is inflated. In some cases, a device called a stent (wire-mesh tubing in picture) is also placed at the site of narrowing or blockage in order to keep the artery open.

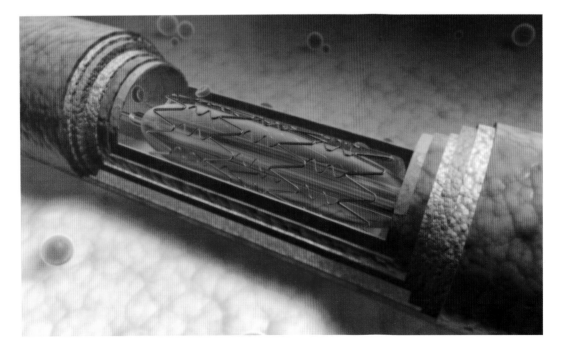

LAMINECTOMY

Laminectomy is an operation on the spine that removes a thin piece of bone from one or more vertebrae. This piece of bone, called the lamina (plural: laminae), forms part of the protective arch that covers the spinal cord and runs over the root of a spinal nerve. Removing the lamina helps to widen a spinal canal that has become narrowed as a result of age-related, degenerative changes.

WHY LAMINECTOMY IS NEEDED

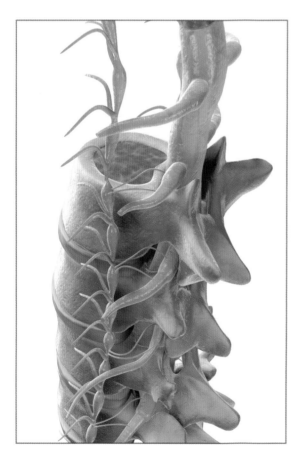

BELOW Diagram of a normal vertebral column showing disks, vertebrae, spinal nerve roots, and spinal cord.

Known as spinal stenosis, this is associated with enlargement of the facet joints between the vertebrae, which increases pressure on the spinal nerve roots. Narrowing of the spinal canal from other conditions, such as osteoarthritis, osteoporotic fractures, and tumors, can also increase pressure on the spinal cord itself, causing a variety of unpleasant symptoms *(see page 117)*. Laminectomy may be needed for surgical access to an intervertebral disk that has bulged out of place (herniated) to press on the spinal cord. This is often referred to as a "slipped" or "ruptured" disk. Operations to change the shape of a deformed spine will also involve laminectomy as part of the procedure.

The spinal column is made up of 33 small bones (vertebrae) that surround and protect the spinal cord. At the base of the spine, the five sacral vertebrae are fused to form the sacrum, and the four coccygeal vertebrae are fused into the coccyx (tailbone). In the upper part of the spine, the seven cervical (neck), 12 thoracic, and five lumbar vertebrae interlock in a series of sliding joints that give your backbone flexibility. These upper 24 vertebrae are separated from each other by the intervertebral disks. These are pads of cartilage which have a tough, flexible outer coat (the annulus fibrosis) and a soft, jelly-like center (the nucleus pulposus). They are designed to act as shock absorbers, cushioning the vertebrae from sudden jolts.

- **Can it be done as an outpatient?** No. Admission to hospital is necessary.

- **Do I need a general anesthetic?** Yes.

- **What special tests are needed?** Diagnosis is usually made on symptoms and examination. Plain X-ray and myelography (in which a special dye is injected in a region [subarachnoid space] surrounding the spinal cord to outline it on X-ray) may be carried out. Magnetic resonance imaging (MRI) or computed tomography (CT) scans are also employed to identify if a disk is injured, or if spinal cord compression is present. Electromyography, a test that measures nerve impulses to muscles, may also be suggested.

- **How long does the surgery take?** From 30 minutes to one hour.

- **What is the mortality rate?** Around one in 500 (0.2%)

- **How long will I be in hospital?** Patients usually stay in hospital for an average of two to three days.

- **How expensive is it?** $ $

- **How many are performed in the US each year?** Around 230,000 laminectomies are performed in the US each year. Just over half of patients (53%) are male. There is a trend toward inpatient procedures becoming less common as more non-surgical alternatives and minimal spinal surgical operations become available. Over 860,000 outpatient procedures, including injections, are carried out annually to treat intervertebral disk disorders.

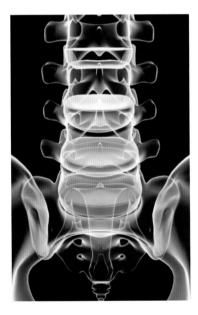

ABOVE A diagram showing the position of the intervertebral disks (in red).

With increasing age, the intervertebral disks start to wear out, dehydrate, stiffen, and shrink so they are more susceptible to damage. This can weaken the protective, fibrous outer coat, so that the soft center (nucleus pulposus) bulges through under pressure. If it bulges forward, it may not cause any symptoms. If it bulges backward, however, it protrudes into the spinal canal and may press on the root of a spinal nerve, or on the spinal cord itself, to cause symptoms *(see below)*. Laminectomy allows surgical access to the disk so that it can be removed or reshaped as part of a lumbar diskectomy.

Factors that increase the chance of a disk herniating include improper lifting of heavy loads, smoking cigarettes, being overweight, and performing repetitive strenuous activities.

Symptoms

Symptoms due to pressure on the spinal cord or spinal nerves (due to stenosis or a prolapsed intervertebral disk) can include:

- Back pain, which can be severe enough to cause immobility.
- Pains shooting down the leg (sciatica) or arm if a cervical disk is involved.
- Leg pain on walking (claudication).
- Weakness, numbness, or tingling sensations in one or both legs, arms, or a buttock.
- Burning sensations in the spine, shoulders, neck, or arm.
- Difficulty with, or loss of, bladder or bowel control.

LAMINECTOMY
STEP-BY-STEP

EMERGENCY OR PLANNED LAMINECTOMY

Some open laminectomies are emergency procedures to relieve sudden pressure on the spinal cord (e.g. from a tumor) that might lead to paralysis. Most are planned procedures, however, for persistent or deteriorating symptoms such as pain, numbness, or tingling in the limbs. Most disk herniations (90%) occur in the lower spine between the 4th and 5th lumbar vertebrae (L4–L5), or between the 5th lumbar vertebra and the sacrum (L5–S1). In the thorax, the level that is most likely to be affected is between the 8th and 12th thoracic vertebrae. In the neck, a herniated disk is most likely to occur between the 5th and 6th or the 4th and 5th cervical vertebrae.

After being anesthetized, you will usually be positioned face down on the operating table, or sometimes on your side.

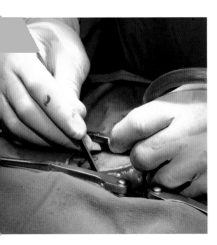

❶ The surgeon makes a 2 in to 5 in (5 cm to 12 cm) cut down the middle of the spine over the affected region of the back. The cut is deepened and the muscles (erector spinae) which run vertically down either side of the spine are scraped away from the vertebrae to expose the underlying bone.

ABOVE After making an incision, the surgeon carefully removes muscle remnants that would hinder bone removal during a laminectomy.

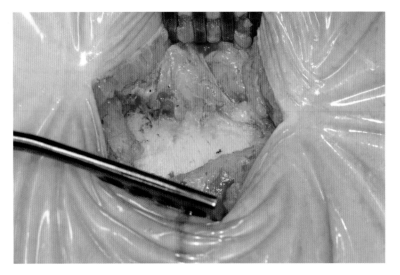

RIGHT Clamps hold the incision open during spinal surgery.

Artificial disk prosthesis

If the spine is otherwise healthy, an artificial disk replacement may be inserted during an operation (anterior lumbar diskectomy) to remove a disk in the lower lumbar region. An incision is made in the lower abdomen and the abdominal contents moved to one side. The surgeon moves the large blood vessels covering the spine out of the way to expose the lower lumbar vertebrae. The herniated disk is then removed, the disk space is cleaned, and an artificial disk prosthesis inserted. A similar procedure can be carried out in the neck to insert an artificial cervical disk.

Microdiskectomy

Microsurgery is performed through a small 1 in to 1.5 in (2.5 cm to 3.5 cm) incision over the spine. The erector spinae muscles are moved to one side, and the surgeon enters the spinal canal by removing a membrane (ligamentum flavum) that covers the spinal nerve roots. Using an operating microscope or special magnifying glasses (loupes), the surgeon removes a small part of one of the facet joints between two vertebrae to relieve pressure over the nerve. The nerve root is then gently moved to one side and the part of the intervertebral disk pressing on it is cut away. This procedure does not remove the lamina(e). This procedure is most effective for treating leg pain (radiculopathy) due to a disk pressing on a lumbar nerve root, rather than back pain. It can be performed as a day case or with just one overnight stay in hospital.

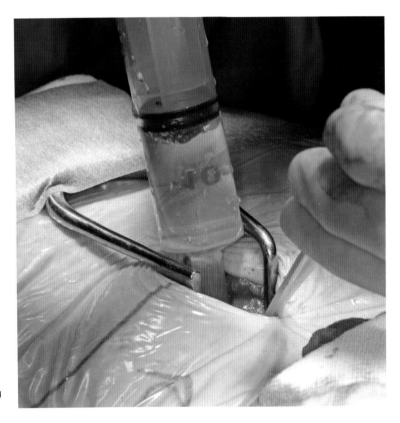

RIGHT A surgeon uses saline (salt) solution to wash away blood and improve vision during spinal surgery.

❷ The surgeon will identify the correct laminae to remove by counting down the vertebrae from a fixed point, or by taking an intra-operative X-ray. The surgeon nibbles away at the lamina(e) to be removed using a variety of special bone cutters. If performing a diskectomy, very little bone needs to be removed to expose the part of the disk to be cut away.

❸ If performing an operation to decompress the spine (for example because of narrowing from osteoarthritis or a tumor), a lot of bone may need to be removed. The surgeon may excise the spinous process in the center of the vertebral arch, as well as the laminae on either side. He or she may also trim the underside of the facet joints, between the vertebrae, to give the nerve roots more room.

REMOVING DAMAGED TISSUES

❹ The surgeon clears away any bone fragments that are pressing on the nerve root (e.g. osteophytes — which are small bony outgrowths that can develop as part of osteoarthritis) and may also remove a membrane (ligamentum flavum) that covers the nerve root. If removal of a herniated intervertebral disk is necessary because it has ruptured into the spinal canal, the outer coat (annulus fibrosis) is cut and the inner nucleus pulposus is removed. In simple cases, this procedure (diskectomy) can be carried out on its own using new minimally invasive techniques without the need for laminectomy *(see page 121)*.

RIGHT **Close-up of an exposed spinal cord (center) with screws inserted to stabilize the vertebral bones on either side.**

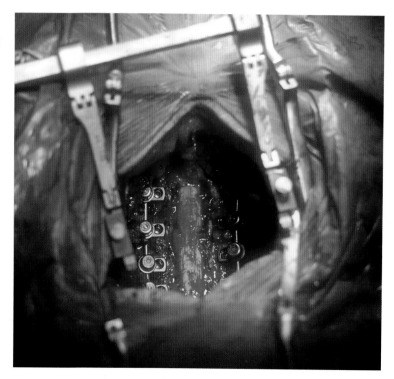

BELOW **Staples are used to close the wound after spinal surgery.**

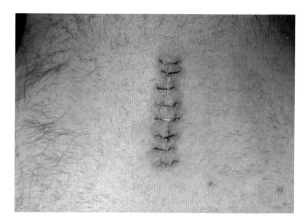

❺ If a lot of bone is removed from the spine, it may become unstable. The surgeon may therefore carry out a spinal fusion. Neighboring vertebrae are joined and stabilized using metal rods *(see above)*, or by inserting a bone graft removed from the hip bone. This heals to fuse the bones together and stabilize the spine. Fusion is usually recommended following a neck (cervical) diskectomy, although there is currently a move toward inserting an artificial disk prosthesis instead.

❻ After completing the operation, any bleeding points are carefully sealed, and the muscles moved back and sewn into place. The skin wound is then closed using stitches or staples *(see left)*, depending on surgeon choice.

LATEST TECHNIQUES

One of the latest advances to this procedure is a form of percutaneous diskectomy *(see box below)* called DISC Nucleoplasty. An imaging technique guides the placing of a needle into the center of the herniated disk. A probe is then inserted that uses a form of plasma energy (coblation) to heat tissues to 104–158 °F (40–70 °C). This destroys part of the disk to create a channel. A series of around six channels are made during the procedure, depending on the amount of tissue reduction required.

You can usually go home on the same day that you have a routine percutaneous diskectomy. You will be advised to avoid bending, twisting, lifting, and prolonged sitting. As the surgeon does not directly remove the herniated disk, there is no guarantee that this procedure will reduce pressure on a spinal nerve or improve symptoms.

BELOW Intra-operative CT scanning helps to guide the surgeon during spinal surgery.

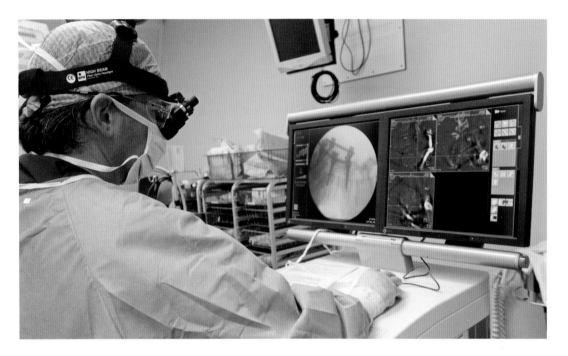

Minimally invasive diskectomy

The center of a prolapsed disk can be removed, or decompressed, through a small needle (cannula) inserted into the back, through the skin. This is called percutaneous diskectomy and can be performed under local anesthesia and sedation, or a general anesthetic. The needle is inserted under guidance using imaging techniques such as X-ray or fluoroscopy. Special tools are then used to remove the nucleus pulposus either by cutting it out, sucking it out, or evaporating it with lasers.

This is an ideal outpatient technique for patients in whom the outer wall of the intervertebral disk is intact (not ruptured). It is usually carried out if pain remains severe, despite four or more weeks of non-surgical treatment, or if there are signs of nerve damage, such as weakness or loss of feeling in a limb. It cannot be carried out if MRI or CT scans show that part of the disk has ruptured into the spinal canal, or where there is narrowing of the spinal canal (spinal stenosis).

LAMINECTOMY
QUESTIONS & ANSWERS

What are the benefits?

Open laminectomy can relieve pain, tingling, numbness, and other symptoms associated with compression of the spinal nerve roots and spinal cord.

What are the risks?

As well as the general risks associated with surgery and general anesthesia *(see pages 10–11)*, back surgery can result in a leak of cerebrospinal fluid due to a tear in the membranes covering the spinal cord. This occurs in 1% to 2% of cases, and is treated by lying still for one or two days until the leak seals. There is also a risk of nerve or spinal cord damage, which could result in bowel or bladder incontinence, or even paralysis, although this is rare. The risks associated with surgery in the lower (lumbar) part of the back are relatively small, especially if performed because of a herniated disk. The risks associated with surgery in the more delicate neck (cervical) and thoracic regions are higher, especially if surgery is needed because of osteoarthritis, osteoporosis, or a tumor in which the anatomy may be abnormal, or the bones more crumbly than usual. High risk operations are normally only carried out if essential to prevent paralysis. Other risks include persistent pain and re-occurrence of the problem, such as a herniated disk.

Are there any alternatives?

Symptoms due to a slipped disk may improve over six to 12 weeks as swelling subsides. Conservative treatments include hot or cold compresses, physiotherapy exercises, spinal manipulation (including chiropractic or osteopathy), traction (rare nowadays), painkillers (oral drugs, injections, or sometimes an epidural or selective nerve block), and antispasmodic drugs. Injection of a steroid drug into the epidural space around a painful nerve root can reduce inflammation, swelling, and pain.

Treatment with a special injection that dissolves part of the disk may be possible *(see page 121)*.

Older people with spinal stenosis may have an Interspinous Process Decompression System inserted. This is a titanium implant which is inserted into the back of the lumbar spine. It prevents the patient bending too far backward at the narrowed part of the spine, and can reduce leg pain and low back pain.

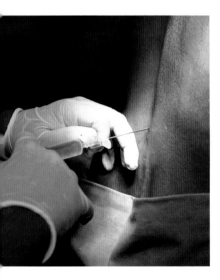

BELOW An anesthesiologist injects local anesthetic into a patient's lower back.

Glucosamine

Glucosamine sulfate is needed in the body for the formation of cartilage and taking glucosamine supplements may prove helpful for people with a prolapsed intervertebral disk.

What can I do to prepare?

Avoid excess stress which can make you subconsciously tense your back muscles and can worsen back pain. Try to lose any excess weight. If you smoke, do your utmost to stop. Exercise regularly to strengthen abdominal and spinal muscles. Improve your posture — keep your spine straight when walking and avoid slouching your shoulders.

Sit correctly: keep square on the chair with your bottom well back and your spine upright; use chair arms to take some weight off your shoulders and lower back. Wear flat or low shoes, not high heels. Sleep on a comfortable mattress that is not overly hard or soft, and use only one pillow.

What if I don't have the operation?

Pain may worsen without treatment, but in the case of a herniated disk can get better. Some conditions, such as spinal canal narrowing (stenosis), that cause progressive pressure on the spinal cord or spinal nerve roots, may result in permanent nerve damage, weakness, numbness, and even paralysis if surgery is not performed.

What happens during the recovery period?

Your blood pressure, pulse, limb movements, and nerve sensation will be monitored at regular intervals. Pain relief is provided by injections

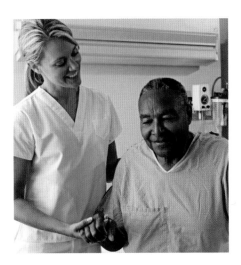

or you may have a pump that releases pain relief (patient controlled analgesia) when you need it. You may be encouraged to mobilize as soon as possible. It is important that you pass urine regularly on your own as this shows that the nerves involved have not been damaged during surgery. Visible stitches and clips are taken out ten to 12 days following surgery. You can usually return to work after four to six weeks if your job does not involve lifting or prolonged sitting. You may be advised not to drive for six weeks, and to avoid driving for longer than 30 minutes initially. You should avoid bending, twisting, lifting, and prolonged sitting for as long as your surgeon advises.

LEFT Patients are encouraged to become mobile soon after surgery.

Learning to lift

Recurrent backache can often be prevented by learning the correct way to lift:

• Stand close to the load, feet on either side of it.

• Squat down by bending at the knees and hips, keeping your back straight and upright.

• Keep your elbows tucked in and grasp the object with both your hands (not your fingers).

• Lean forward slightly and, in one smooth action, straighten your hips and knees while lifting the object and holding it close.

• To lower a heavy load, reverse this action, keeping your back straight at all times.

• Never combine bending and lifting.

CAROTID ENDARTERECTOMY

Carotid endarterectomy is a surgical procedure in which one of the carotid arteries is cut open and cleaned. The left and right carotid arteries carry blood up through the neck to the brain. Like other arteries in the body, these can become hardened and narrowed as a result of atherosclerosis, in which a sticky build-up of cholesterol and calcium forms on their inner walls (see page 125). This causes a partial blockage, usually where the larger common carotid artery divides and narrows to form the internal carotid arteries (which supply the brain) and external carotid arteries (which supply the face and scalp). Carotid endarterectomy is designed to clear this blockage and reduce the risk of a stroke.

WHAT IS A STROKE?

A stroke is a sudden loss of control of one or more body functions due to an interruption in the blood supply to part of the brain. This can result from a ruptured blood vessel that bleeds into the brain or, more commonly, when a clot blocks a blood vessel cutting off blood supply to a variable number of brain cells. When a clot forms within the brain, this type of stroke is classed as a cerebral thrombosis. When the clot forms elsewhere in the body and travels to the brain, it is called a cerebral embolism.

Clogging of the carotid arteries increases the risk of a stroke due to restricted blood flow, as well as cerebral embolism, which may be prevented by carotid endarterectomy. Unfortunately, the operation itself

Symptoms of a stroke

Symptoms vary, depending on the part of the brain affected, and the number of brain cells that die.
A stroke may produce:
- Sudden unconsciousness or collapse.
- Confusion or loss of memory.
- An inability to move part of the body on one side, such as the left arm and left leg.
- Weakness on one side of the face with drooping of the mouth or eye.

- Difficulty with speech.
- Difficulty swallowing.
- Difficulty understanding words or finding the right word.
- Visual disturbances, including double vision.
- Vomiting.

The effects usually come on quickly and may get worse over a period of several hours.

CAROTID ENDARTERECTOMY AT A GLANCE

• *Can it be done as an outpatient?* No. Admission to hospital is necessary.

• *Do I need a general anesthetic?* Usually, yes, but it can be performed under a local anesthetic and sedation if your surgeon thinks this will suit you better. This means that surgery can still be performed on someone who also has lung or heart disease, for example, and who is less likely to tolerate a general anesthetic. Local anesthesia also allows the surgeon to talk to you and assess the effects of reduced blood flow to the brain during surgery.

• *What special tests are needed?* A doctor may recognize the presence of carotid narrowing by listening to your carotid arteries with a stethoscope to hear noises caused by turbulent blood flow. The state of your carotid arteries, and the amount of blood flow through them, is assessed using tests such as ultrasound scanning, a magnetic resonance angiography (MRA), computed tomographic angiography (CTA), or a special X-ray that uses a dye to outline the blood vessels (arteriography or angiography). This allows the doctor to assess whether narrowing is mild (less than 50%), moderate (50% to 69%), or severe (70% to 99%). Surgery is usually recommended once carotid artery narrowing is classed as severe.

• *How long does the surgery take?* Usually around two hours or less.

• *What is the mortality rate?* Less than one in 260 (0.38%).

• *How long will I be in hospital?* Patients usually stay in hospital for an average of two to three days.

• *How expensive is it?* 💲💲

• *How many are performed in the US each year?* Around 115,000 operations are performed in the US each year, 70% of which are in people aged 65 years or older. There are slightly more male (57%) than female patients.

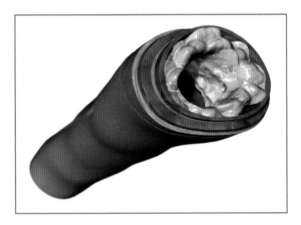

also carries a risk of stroke, as it may dislodge a clot to produce a new embolus. Surgery is therefore only recommended for people with a high chance of developing a stroke within the next few years.

A carotid endarterectomy is especially indicated for people experiencing mini-strokes, which are also known as transient ischemic attacks.

LEFT Diagram showing an artery clogged with plaque.

WHAT ARE TIAS?

Transient ischemic attacks (TIAs) are similar to a stroke but, by definition, symptoms totally resolve within 24 hours. They can also cause fleeting darkening or loss of vision (known medically as amaurosis fugax). TIAs are often recurrent and occur when clumps of blood cell fragments (platelets) lodge in small blood vessels within the brain. This temporarily blocks the circulation to some brain cells to produce symptoms. The platelet clots break up and clear before brain cells die from lack of blood, so that symptoms disappear within 24 hours.

Carotid Endarterectomy Step-by-step

Clearing a blocked carotid artery

The platelet clots that cause TIAs are an important warning sign that a stroke may occur in the future. Five years on, at least one in six sufferers will have experienced a full-blown stroke. When the clots are identified as coming from a clogged carotid artery, carotid endarterectomy or carotid angioplasty *(see page 129)* have the potential to solve the problem and prevent a stroke from occurring. Research suggests that surgery to treat severe carotid stenosis can halve the risk of experiencing a stroke over the next five to eight years. It is most effective when carried out within two weeks of a TIA or stroke. If both carotid arteries are blocked and require endarterectomy, this is usually carried out as two separate procedures.

If performed under a general anesthetic, you will receive drugs via a drip to put you to sleep. If having the procedure under a local anesthetic, a numbing agent is injected into the skin of your neck. More local anesthetic can be injected during the procedure if you feel uncomfortable. You will be given a sedative too, so you are less likely to remember the operation afterward.

The anesthesiologist may insert a special drip into an artery in your wrist to allow careful monitoring of your blood pressure during and after the operation. This is because blood pressure is partly controlled by special sensors (baroreceptors), some of which are found within the internal carotid arteries. They monitor the pressure of blood going to the brain. If this pressure reduces during surgery, the sensors may trigger changes which need to be controlled.

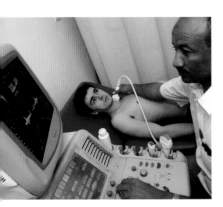

ABOVE A technician uses ultrasound to examine the carotid artery of a patient for any abnormalities, such as stenosis (narrowing).

RIGHT A colored angiogram of the left carotid artery (yellow) in a patient's neck. Severe stenosis (narrowing) is reducing blood flow (lower center).

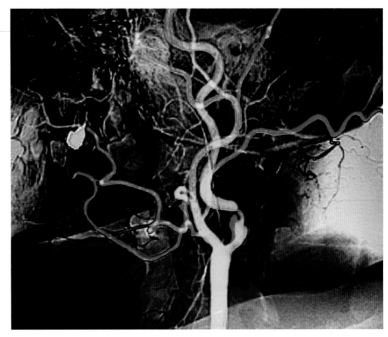

❶ The surgeon makes a cut that runs obliquely for 2.75 in to 4 in (7 cm to 10 cm) from the angle of your jaw toward your breastbone. This exposes the common carotid artery and its branches.

❷ The affected part of the carotid artery, and its branches, are clamped off. During the procedure, your brain will continue to receive blood from the carotid artery on the other side, and from the vertebral arteries. To ensure your brain receives an uninterrupted blood supply, however, the surgeon may insert a shunt (plastic tube) above and below the area of repair to form a bypass, so blood continues traveling up to the internal carotid artery on the affected side. If you are having the operation under local anesthesia and sedation, the surgeon may wake you from time to time and test your brain function by asking a simple question and asking you to move your hand. If your responses are slow, the surgeon may insert the shunt at that stage.

BELOW A colored 3D CT scan of an atheroma plaque (orange, rippled) in the internal carotid artery in the neck.

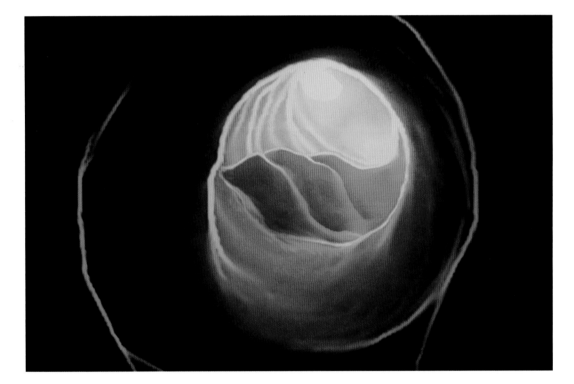

Blood supply to the brain

The blood supply to the brain arrives through four arteries. Two vertebral arteries enter the skull from the back and mainly supply the brainstem and cerebellum. The two internal carotid arteries enter the skull from the front of the neck and mainly supply the two cerebral hemispheres. All four arteries usually join up to form a circuit called the Circle of Willis. This helps to maintain an adequate supply of blood to all parts of the brain if one artery becomes blocked. The effectiveness of this circle of arteries varies from person to person and it often does not protect people from the symptoms of a stroke if one of the arteries becomes blocked by an embolus.

❸ The main trunk of the artery is then opened lengthwise. The inner lining of the artery, and the material (plaque) that has accumulated on it, are carefully removed to expose a new, healthy, smooth, pale pink lining. If the underlying tissue is diseased, however, a section of the artery may be removed and replaced with an artificial graft.

RIGHT An opened artery showing plaque (in this case in the aorta, a large artery that arises in the heart).

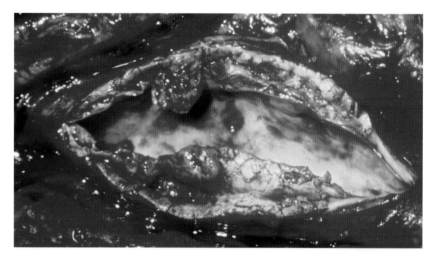

RIGHT A surgeon prepares to remove plaque from a clogged artery (in this case, in the aorta).

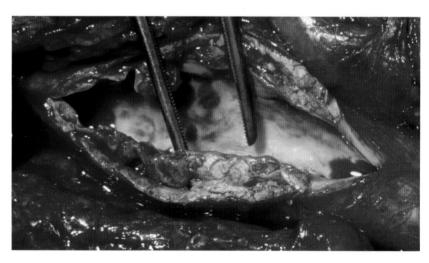

❹ Once the surgeon is happy that blood can flow through the repaired artery without obstruction, the artery is closed using very fine stitches. Usually, the surgeon inserts a patch into the artery wall and stitches it in place to widen the vessel and significantly reduce the chance of future re-stenosis (narrowing). If a patch is used, this may be formed from a short length of vein taken from the leg, or the surgeon may use a special sheet of synthetic material.

❺ The clamps or bypass shunt are now removed and the surgeon checks for any areas of bleeding, which are repaired. Sometimes a drainage tube is placed in the neck to prevent a build-up of blood. This will be removed when it stops draining, one or two days later.

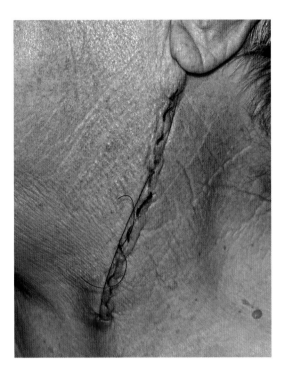

6 The skin incision is closed using dissolvable stitches or staple clips that are removed around five days after the operation *(see left)*.

LEFT A healing scar, 12 days after a carotid endarterectomy.

Carotid angioplasty

A relatively new procedure, called carotid stenting or carotid angioplasty, is a less invasive way of treating carotid narrowing than endarterectomy. A narrow, flexible tube (catheter) with a small balloon and wire-mesh tubing (stent) on one end, is inserted into the femoral artery in the groin under local anesthetic. The catheter is advanced through the circulation, without blocking blood flow, until its tip reaches the carotid artery. When it reaches the area of narrowing, the balloon is inflated which opens the stent. This presses against the area of narrowing, compressing the plaque and keeping the artery open to improve blood flow *(see above right)*. As with endarterectomy, there is a small risk (1% to 3%) of causing a stroke during the procedure by knocking off a piece of debris to cause a cerebral embolism. It is therefore only recommended for people with severe stenosis in which the risks of a stroke occurring naturally are higher than the risk of surgery. As it is less invasive than endarterectomy, you usually only stay in hospital overnight and can return to normal activities as soon as you feel ready. The long-term benefits, and risk of re-stenosis, are not yet clear.

A ten year follow-up of people who had undergone either stenting or endarterectomy showed both groups had a similar risk of stroke within 30 days of the procedure, but ultrasound showed that re-narrowing of the carotid artery was more likely to occur within one year in those having the stenting operation (27%) than in those having endarterectomy (18%). Those who smoked had more than three times the risk of re-stenosis than non-smokers.

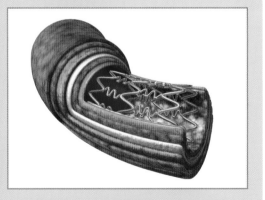

ABOVE A stent may be inserted during angioplasty to open up a narrowed carotid artery.

Carotid Endarterectomy
Questions & Answers

What are the benefits?

Carotid endarterectomy can prevent TIAs and may stop you experiencing a stroke. The National Institute of Neurological Disorders and Stroke estimated that, in people who have already experienced a stroke, surgery can reduce the risk of experiencing another within two years from 25% to less than 10%.

What are the risks?

As well as the general risks associated with surgery and general anesthesia *(see pages 10–11)*, carotid endarterectomy carries a risk of causing a stroke during the operation. This risk is between one and three per 100 people having surgery. The surgeon will only have recommended that you have the procedure if he or she believes that your risk of experiencing a stroke without surgery is higher than that associated with the operation. There is also a small risk of complications such as a heart attack or kidney failure. Rarely, surgery may cause damage to nerves in the neck that pass close to the carotid artery, which may mean you develop numbness on one side of the face, a hoarse voice, or weakness of muscles in the tongue, lower jaw, or neck, which may affect speech. These nerve problems usually improve within a month without any special treatment. The carotid artery can re-narrow enough to require further surgery, a risk that is especially high in smokers.

Are there any alternatives?

TIAs are treated by taking a drug that lowers platelet stickiness (e.g. aspirin) which can often prevent a stroke from occurring.

What can I do to prepare?

Try to keep as healthy as possible *(see page 131)*.

What if I don't have the operation?

If you don't have the operation, your symptoms will continue and may worsen. A surgeon only recommends the procedure when he or she believes your risk of experiencing a stroke without treatment is higher than the risks of the operation itself.

What happens during the recovery period?

You will usually be taken to an intensive care or high dependency unit for up to 24 hours so that you can be monitored closely. You may experience some swelling of the neck which usually settles within ten days. Regular gentle exercise is recommended to help your recovery but you should avoid vigorous exercise for six weeks. You can usually start driving within three weeks, once you can perform an emergency stop safely. Return to work is usually within one month, depending on the nature of your job. You will usually continue with a low dose of blood thinning medication, such as aspirin, to reduce unwanted blood clot formation. If you notice any changes in your ability to think straight (cognitive function) or severe headaches, tell your doctor immediately.

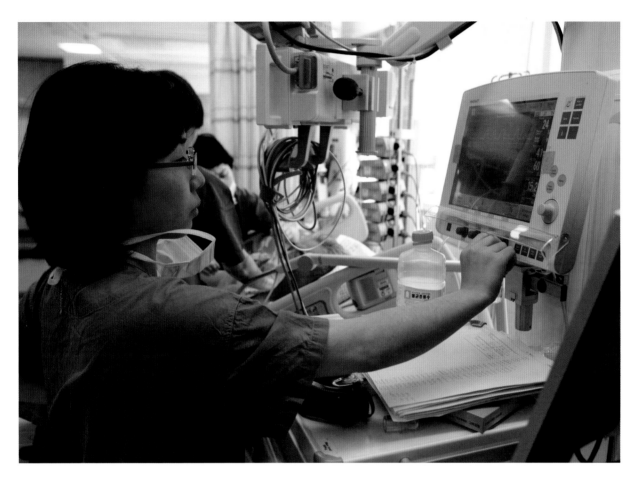

ABOVE A patient recovering from an operation is monitored in an intensive care unit.

Lifestyle modifications

To help avoid a stroke:

- If you smoke, do your utmost to stop.
- Try to lose any excess weight.
- Exercise regularly, at least 30 minutes per day and preferably more.
- Keep your alcohol intake within the recommended safe limits.
- Your doctor is likely to prescribe a blood cholesterol-lowering medication, such as a statin drug; in this case, consider also taking co-enzyme Q10 supplements to maintain your energy levels and help reduce muscle side effects related to statin drugs.
- If you have diabetes, ensure that your blood glucose levels are always well controlled.
- If you have high blood pressure, it is important to ensure this is well-controlled with medication.

LAPAROSCOPY AND LAPAROTOMY

Laparotomy (from the Greek, laparos, meaning soft) is a term used to describe an incision through the soft part of the abdominal wall, between the ribs and pelvis. The term is also used to mean an exploration of the abdomen. At one time laparotomy was a common procedure to confirm a diagnosis and the extent of disease, especially when the cause of abdominal symptoms was uncertain. It is now less common, thanks to the development of diagnostic techniques, such as ultrasound, computed tomography (CT), magnetic resonance imaging (MRI), and positron emission tomography (PET), which allow diagnoses to be made before resorting to surgery. It is also less common as a result of minimal access procedures, such as endoscopy and laparoscopy.

WHAT ARE ADHESIONS?

Laparoscopy is often referred to as keyhole surgery. It allows a surgeon to explore the internal organs with a viewing device, and to operate using surgical instruments inserted through a variable number of small incisions. Carbon dioxide gas is pumped into the abdominal cavity to expand the space and improve the view. As most diseases of the gut involve its lining, however, laparoscopy does not replace endoscopic examination through viewing devices inserted via the mouth or anus.

One of the most common reasons for laparotomy or laparoscopy is to divide abdominal adhesions (adhesiolysis).

Adhesions are strands of fibrous, scar tissue that form within body cavities as part of the healing process. They may form thin sheets of tissue, like shrink-wrap, or resemble thick, non-elastic bands. Adhesions can form a web of matting over the surface of internal organs, causing them

Symptoms of adhesions

Symptoms that can be due to adhesions include:

- Abdominal pain.
- Bloating.
- Small bowel obstruction.
- Painful intercourse.
- Reduced fertility.
- Pelvic pain.

Adhesions can also form within the chest, around the heart. Having adhesions adds an estimated 24 minutes to the total time of an abdominal or pelvic operation, as they obscure the normal anatomy and careful dissection is needed to separate organs that are stuck together.

LAPAROSCOPY AND LAPAROTOMY AT A GLANCE

- **Can it be done as an outpatient?** No. Admission to hospital is necessary.

- **Do I need a general anesthetic?** Yes.

- **What special tests are needed?** Diagnosis of adhesions is based on symptoms and clinical examination. A rectal examination is performed to detect any tenderness or swellings in the pelvis. In women an "internal" or pelvic examination is also needed. Blood tests are performed to look for signs of infection (high white blood cell count) and, in women of fertile age, a pregnancy test is important to exclude ectopic pregnancy. Adhesions are usually diagnosed during laparoscopy or laparotomy. They do not show up well on X-ray or ultrasound. CT and MRI scans may help to determine the extent of adhesion-related problems, such as small bowel obstruction.

- **How long does the surgery take?** Laparotomy and laparoscopy can take between one and three hours, or more. Duration depends on the reason for surgery, the extent of any adhesions, and whether or not complications develop during surgery, such as perforation of the bowel.

- **What is the mortality rate?** Around one in 70 for emergency inpatient laparoscopy (1.4%). Around one in 40 (2.6%) for division of adhesions. Around one in five (19%) with laparotomy — the rate is high because patients who require emergency laparotomy are usually very sick, often with peritonitis (widespread infection of the abdominal cavity). The highest risk is for infants under the age of one year, and elderly people over the age of 85 years.

- **How long will I be in hospital?** Patients usually stay in hospital for an average of five days for diagnostic laparoscopy; nine to ten days for exploratory laparotomy, and eight to nine days for excision of peritoneal adhesions.

- **How expensive is it?**
  Laparoscopy 💲💲
  Division of peritoneal adhesions 💲💲
  Laparotomy 💲💲💲

- **How many are performed in the US each year?** Diagnostic laparoscopies account for around 13,000 operations, of which over 70% are on female patients. Around 16,300 exploratory laparotomies are performed each year, divided fairly evenly between males and females. Around 88,000 operations are carried out to divide or excise peritoneal adhesions, of which 65% are in women. In addition, 2.5 million outpatient procedures involve the female genital organs, many of which use laparoscopy.

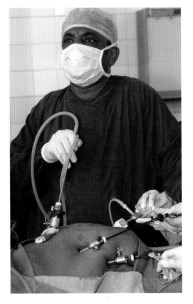

to stick together. The most usual cause is internal cuts and burns made during surgery. Following pelvic or abdominal surgery, 93% of people are found to have adhesions when re-examined at a later date, making them one of the most common post-operative complications. They are especially likely to form in the female pelvis following gynecological surgery. The risk of developing adhesions increases with age, and with the number of operations you undergo. Adhesions start to form within three to five days of surgery. Although they may never cause problems, symptoms can arise months or even years after they originally formed *(see page 132)*. Abdominal adhesions are also found in 10% of people who have never had surgery, as their formation can be triggered by other traumas, such as infection, bleeding, disease processes, chemotherapy, radiotherapy, and reduced blood supply.

LEFT A surgeon performs laparoscopic surgery. The laparoscope is designed to view inside the abdomen through small incisions in the body.

Laparoscopy and Laparotomy
Step-by-step

Laparotomy

Laparotomy may be needed as an exploratory operation in patients who present with severe abdominal pain of unknown cause. It is especially likely if the patient is febrile, vomiting, and showing signs of widespread abdominal infection (peritonitis) or bowel obstruction. Laparotomy allows the surgeon a wide field of view, and instant access to all abdominal and pelvic organs. Where symptoms are more localized, and where a diagnosis such as appendicitis *(see page 92)* or ectopic pregnancy is suspected, the surgeon may first attempt to solve the problem using laparoscopic or minimal access techniques. If these are not sufficient, he or she will have no qualms about converting to an open laparotomy operation. This is not seen as a failure of surgical technique, but simply as safe practice.

The surgeon will re-examine your abdomen once you are anesthetized and your muscles are relaxed. He or she may feel a mass that was not detectable before, which helps them decide where to make their laparotomy incision.

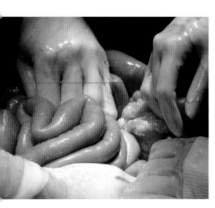

ABOVE Surgeons examine loops of small intestine during an exploratory laparotomy.

❶ The incision most commonly used for laparotomy is a vertical one, down the center of the abdomen, just to the left or right of the midline, swerving around the belly button. It is positioned more above or below the umbilicus, depending on the probable site of problems. As this incision passes through a tough sheet of tissue (aponeurosis) that is relatively free from blood vessels, it minimizes bleeding and is quicker to create and close. Other vertical incisions are possible, as are a variety of transverse and oblique incisions, depending on the access needed.

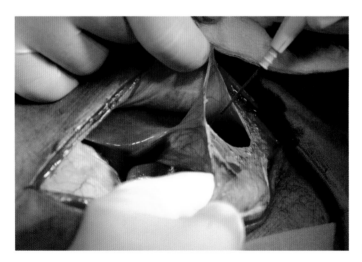

LEFT Incision for laparotomy.

Re-opening the abdomen

If a patient has previously had surgery, the surgeon may use the old incision line if it is in a suitable site. This is especially helpful for dissecting off old adhesions, especially if extended slightly beyond the old incision. It also allows an ugly or stretched scar to be removed (as an elongated ellipse) and refashioned to achieve a better cosmetic outcome.

2 After cutting the skin, and underlying subcutaneous fat, the three layers of the abdominal wall (containing the external oblique, internal oblique, and transverse muscles) are also cut, split, or displaced in line with the vertical skin incision. Any bleeding points are sealed with heat (diathermy), taking care not to burn the skin. Large cut blood vessels may need to be tied closed with a fine absorbable suture.

3 The assistant holds the edges of the wound firmly open, and the surgeon carefully picks up a fold of peritoneal membrane with toothed forceps. After ensuring no bowel is attached (very likely if re-opening an old scar), he or she makes an incision in the membrane to enter the abdominal cavity. Any visible pus is swabbed and sent to the laboratory for microscopy and culture. This helps to identify the organism involved and the antibiotics to which they are sensitive.

BELOW Clamps are applied to cut tissues.

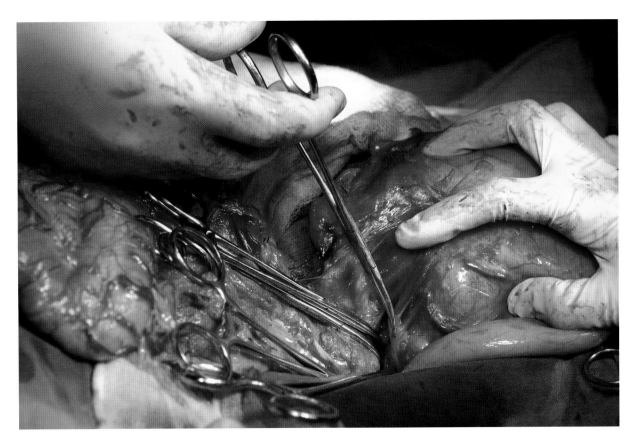

Assessing all the abdominal organs

At some stage during the operation, the surgeon will carefully examine all the abdominal organs by feel and, where possible, by sight *(see opposite above)*. The examination is carried out in a methodical order using the same sequence so nothing is missed. This helps to identify the cause of present symptoms, and unforeseen diseases of the liver, gallbladder, stomach, kidneys, pancreas, small intestines, large bowel, and pelvic organs. Sometimes a routine appendectomy is performed *(see page 92)*.

DIVIDING ADHESIONS

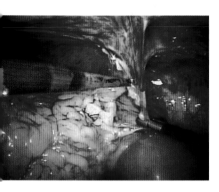

ABOVE A surgeon divides
adhesions during laparoscopic
surgery.

BELOW Clamps hold cut tissues
together as staples are inserted
to close the wound.

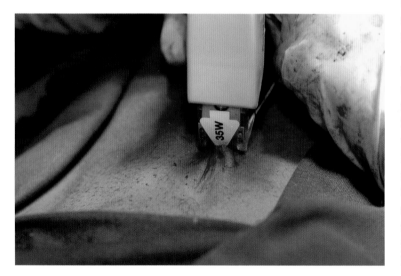

❹ If adhesions are present, these are carefully lifted with tissue-holding forceps to determine the degree to which they are fixed to surrounding structures. Dense adhesions are cut first, followed by those that are more thin and filmy, so that underlying organs are progressively exposed. This is an arduous and hazardous task. The surgeon always clearly identifies what he is cutting before it is cut with a scalpel, scissors, or hot blade (diathermy). He or she never cuts what cannot be seen. When necessary, the table may be rotated so the patient rolls slightly to one side, or the table is positioned head down. This helps organs fall away, under gravity, to improve access. If steep tilts are anticipated, the patient is strapped to the table beforehand. Organs are held out of the way by retractors or packed behind moist swabs.

❺ If the surgeon damages a structure that is firmly stuck to adhesions (for example, by perforating a loop of small bowel), the extent of damage is assessed and repaired at that point, and then checked at the end of the operation. Prompt use of the sucker and gauze swabs helps to minimize contamination of the wound with intestinal contents. Having divided as many adhesions as possible — especially those that form thick, fleshy bands that can constrict organs — the bowel is carefully replaced in such a way as to prevent kinking and reduce the future formation of hernias.

❻ Once all bleeding has stopped, and the surgeon has checked that no other procedures are needed, the abdomen may be rinsed out with warm saline or Ringer's lactate *(see page 137)*. A drain may be inserted if it is likely that fluid or blood may build up at the site of surgery. The incision is then closed using the surgeon's preferred method; either layer by layer, or as one simple mass

Laparoscopic adhesiolysis

To divide adhesions laparoscopically, three or four abdominal puncture sites are needed — one in the umbilicus (belly button) to insert the viewing device (laparoscope) and two or three punctures, usually in the lower abdomen, to insert the surgical instruments *(see opposite)*. Grasping forceps are inserted in one cut to hold the adhesions, gently stretch them, and identify their boundaries. Microscissors or a CO_2 laser are inserted in another incision to carefully cut the adhesions. Dense adhesions are severed first, followed by those that are more thin and filmy, so that underlying organs are progressively exposed. Bleeding points are sealed using a laser or heat (electrocautery).

closure except for the skin. Some surgeons do not suture the peritoneum as they believe this may encourage the formation of adhesions. The skin is then closed with stitches or staples, and the wound is dressed.

BELOW A surgeon performing laparoscopic (keyhole) surgery.

Avoiding adhesions during surgery

Although laparoscopy is associated with less adhesion formation than laparotomy, it still carries a substantial risk of adhesion formation. One of the most recently identified triggers is the starch powder used commercially to coat latex surgical gloves so they are easier to put on. Thoroughly washing the gloves for ten minutes, after putting them on, can reduce adhesion formation, but must be done properly. The suggested technique is to use the surgical scrub solution, povidone-iodine, as this binds starch and turns it black (making it easy to recognize when no starch remains), followed by a sterile water rinse. The better option, of course, is for a surgeon to use powder-free gloves. Sewing the peritoneum is another possible cause of adhesion formation, and some surgeons no longer do this routinely. Post-operative adhesions may also be reduced by carefully irrigating the peritoneal cavity with a special solution (Ringer's lactate) before closing the abdomen at the end of surgery. Adhesion-prevention barriers made from cellulose or Gore-Tex have also been developed, which are used to line surfaces where adhesions commonly form to reduce their occurrence.

LAPAROSCOPY AND LAPAROTOMY
QUESTIONS & ANSWERS

What are the benefits?

Division of adhesions can improve associated long-term (chronic) abdominal pain in more than 80% of people who are affected. It can also improve by 40% to 60% the chance of successful conception where the ovaries and Fallopian tubes are entangled.

What are the risks?

As well as the general risks associated with surgery and general anesthesia *(see pages 10–11)*, adhesions that require surgery often reform as the corrective surgery itself can retrigger their formation, although a surgeon can take steps to reduce their formation *(see page 137)*. Adhesions increase the risk of a surgeon accidentally puncturing the bowel during laparotomy by 21%.

Are there any alternatives?

Adhesion-related symptoms often improve on their own, using painkillers, to avoid the need for surgery. If they cause persistent or severe pain, however, are associated with reduced fertility, of if they cause complications such as small bowel obstruction, surgery is needed. The only way to remove or divide adhesions is surgical.

What can I do to prepare?

BELOW Try to lose any excess weight before surgery.

Try to be as fit and healthy as possible. Eat a well balanced diet, and try to lose any excess weight if surgery is elective and you have time. Take regular exercise. If you smoke, do your utmost to stop.

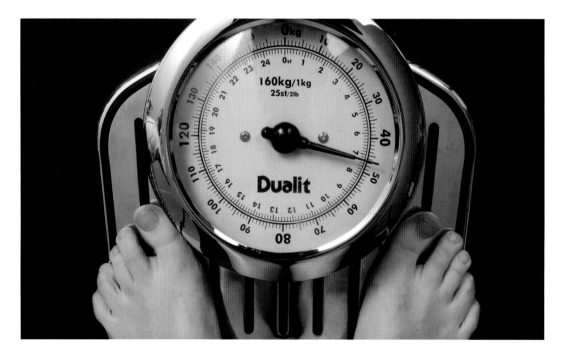

What if I don't have the operation?

If surgery is not carried out when recommended by your surgeon, it is likely that you will experience a worsening of your symptoms. In some cases, laparoscopy or laparotomy are vital to make or confirm the cause of abdominal symptoms, especially if they are due to adhesions.

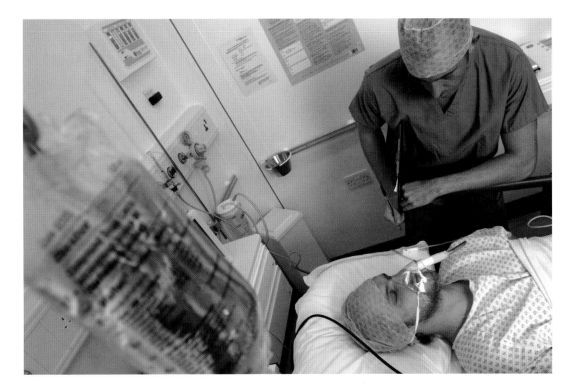

What happens during the recovery period?

After laparotomy, you will have a number of tubes coming from your body, which may include an intravenous infusion (drip), bladder catheter, drainage tubes at the site of operation, a nasogastric tube through the nose to the stomach, and an oxygen source. You may have a pump that releases pain relief (patient controlled analgesia) when you need it. Most of these tubes are removed over the next one to five days. You can start eating and drinking as soon as you feel ready, unless your bowel was punctured and repaired, in which cause you need to wait a few days until your bowel function returns to normal. Visible stitches or clips are removed after seven to 12 days.

Gentle mobilization is important to reduce the risk of deep vein blood clots. You will be advised not to lift anything heavy, or to carry out strenuous activities, for at least the first four to six weeks after a laparotomy, depending on the site and extent of your abdominal wound. You can usually return to work after four to six weeks if your job involves no heavy lifting.

You should not drive until you are advised that you can do so by your doctor and insurance provider. This is usually once you can perform an emergency stop without fear that your wound may hurt.

Transurethral Resection Prostate

Transurethral resection of the prostate (TURP) is an operation to clear the urinary tube (urethra) that runs through the prostate gland. A surgeon inserts a narrow instrument through the end of the penis and pares away, or destroys, excess prostate tissue using a hot wire, microwave heat, or laser energy. This helps to improve male urinary symptoms due to benign prostatic hyperplasia (BPH).

What is the prostate gland?

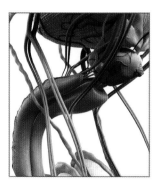

The prostate is a gland that lies just beneath a man's bladder, wrapped around the urethra — the tube through which urine flows from the bladder to the outside world.

The prostate gland secretes a thin, milky fluid that makes up around a third of the male fluids (semen) released during ejaculation. It also contains muscle cells that help the gland to contract.

LEFT A diagram showing the position of the prostate gland. The prostate has a tumor on its posterior wall.

The symptoms of BPH

The symptoms of BPH result from narrowing of the urethra, and from irritation of the bladder as it tries to force urine past the obstruction. Symptoms usually start slowly and become progressively worse.

The obstructive symptoms of prostatism include:
• Straining or difficulty when starting to pass water (hesitancy).
• A weak urinary stream which may start and stop mid-flow.
• Dribbling of urine after voiding.
• Inadequate emptying of the bladder (urinary retention).

The irritative symptoms of prostatism include:
• Having to rush to the toilet (urgency).
• Passing water more often than normal (daytime frequency).
• Having to get up to pass urine at night (nocturia).
• Discomfort when passing water.
• Urinary incontinence.
• A feeling of not having emptied the bladder fully.

Erectile difficulties can also occur, with reduced rigidity of erections, difficulty achieving climax, and discomfort.

Blood in the urine or sperm is not a usual symptom of BPH. If you notice this, tell your doctor as soon as possible as this needs further investigation.

TURP AT A GLANCE

• **Can it be done as an outpatient?** No. Office-based procedures to heat and shrink the prostate are available, however.

• **Do I need a general anesthetic?** TURP is often carried out under spinal or epidural anesthesia *(see page 8)*. General anesthetic can also be used.

• **What special tests are needed?** The size and shape of the prostate gland is assessed by inserting a finger through the anus (digital rectal examination). Urine and blood tests check for infection, kidney function, and may ensure blood clotting time is normal (because of the risk of hemorrhage). Blood levels of the enzyme prostate specific antigen (PSA) *(see page 155)* are measured. Raised levels suggest prostate infection, a markedly enlarged prostate, or a possible prostate cancer. Others tests sometimes needed include urinary flow rate and pressure studies, ultrasound measurement of the prostate gland (using a rectal probe), and residual urinary volume after voiding. Some people have cystoscopy (visual examination of the bladder), and computed tomography or dye X-rays (intravenous pyelogram) to examine the kidneys.

• **How long does the surgery take?** Optimal surgery time is less than 60 minutes. If the prostate is very enlarged, and surgery likely to take longer than 90 minutes, an open prostatectomy *(see page 148)* reduces the risk of complications.

• **What is the mortality rate?** Around 1 in 285 (0.35%)

• **How long will I be in hospital?** Patients usually stay in hospital for an average of three to four days.

• **How expensive is it?** 💲

• **How many are performed in the US each year?** BPH is the most common condition treated by urologists. Around 78,500 TURP operations are performed in the US each year. The development of medical drugs, and other operative techniques, such as transurethral microwave thermotherapy (TUMT) and interstitial laser coagulation (ILC), mean the number of TURPs carried out has slowly declined from the 350,000 carried out per year in the mid-1980s.

BENIGN PROSTATIC HYPERPLASIA (BPH)

After the age of 45, the number of cells in the prostate increases and the gland starts to enlarge. As the prostate gland is wrapped round the urethra, this increased bulk often narrows the urinary outflow. As the prostate enlarges, smooth muscle cells within the prostate also become stretched which triggers a reflex contraction that can further narrow the urethra.

BPH is thought to be triggered by the presence of a hormone, dihydrotestosterone, which forms from the breakdown of the male sex hormone, testosterone. BPH becomes more common with increasing age, so that an estimated 50% of 50-year-olds, 60% of 60-year-olds, 70% of 70-year-olds and so on, develop problems known as "prostatism" or lower urinary tract symptoms (LUTS) *(see page 140)*.

The size of the prostate gland does not necessary relate to severity of symptoms, however. It depends on the direction in which the gland enlarges, and the width of your urinary tube. In some, only a small enlargement in prostate size will squeeze the urethra enough to cause problems. In others, the gland may predominately enlarge outward so that even when it has reached a large size it does not significantly affect urinary flow.

TURP
STEP-BY-STEP

TRANSURETHRAL RESECTION

Although becoming less common, transurethral resection of the prostate using a high-frequency electric arc, or a laser beam, remains the gold-standard surgical treatment for BPH. It is used when medical drugs and less invasive prostate procedures have failed to resolve symptoms of acute, recurrent, or chronic urinary retention. It is also used for men whose prostate is an unusual shape or unusually large, or who have severe lower urinary tract symptoms. Unlike other, less invasive techniques that use microwaves, radio frequency waves, or laser coagulation to heat and shrink the gland, resection removes pieces of prostate tissue that can be examined under a microscope. This helps to rule out the presence of prostate cancer.

❶ The patient is laid on a cystoscopy table with legs raised and apart, and buttocks level with the end of the table. The penis is cleansed with an antiseptic solution. The surgeon carefully examines the urethra, urinary sphincter, prostatic urethra, and the bladder using a narrow viewing device *(see below)*. This identifies any stricture, bladder tumors, or stones, and confirms the patient's individual anatomy. In particular, the surgeon looks for the area in the urethra where the seminal ducts enter. Known as the verumontanum, this landmark helps the surgeon to maintain the correct orientation. Usually, resection is not carried out above this landmark as this risks damaging the external sphincter muscle, and could result in permanent urinary incontinence.

RIGHT A viewing device is inserted into the urethra of a male patient. A laser will also be inserted through the device to treat BPH.

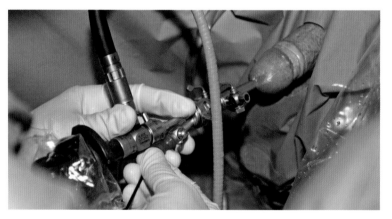

Urethrostomy

If the urethra is too narrow for a viewing device to pass, the surgeon may have to make a cut in the perineum, between the scrotum and anus, to access and cut open the prostatic urethra. This is called a perineal urethrostomy.

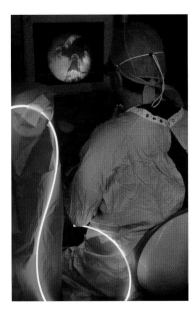

2 The surgeon passes a narrow instrument (endoscope) through the end of the penis. A fiber-optic light and lens system allows the surgeon to directly view the urethra. The surgeon pares away the bulging inner surface of the prostatic urethra where it passes down through the prostate gland. A laser beam *(see left)* or a high-frequency electric arc is used to trim away excess tissue and simultaneously cauterize bleeding points. Cuts are made as the endoscope is withdrawn from the prostate, never when pushing it forward. This cleanly separates the cut tissue from the gland.

3 The surgeon continues to pare away the excess prostate tissue methodically following his or her preferred sequence, dealing first with one lobe then another. The removed tissue is off-white in color and appears granular. The surgeon knows when "healthy" tissue is reached as it appears more smooth, white, and glistening. The average amount of tissue removed during a TURP is 0.8 oz (22 grams), but 1.75 oz (50 grams) or more may be removed if the gland is particularly enlarged.

ABOVE A surgeon uses a greenlight laser to treat BPH.

BELOW A surgeon views the laser vaporization of prostate cells on a monitor as he carefully widens the urethra.

4 Throughout the operation, fluid warmed to body temperature is used to continuously irrigate the urethra at low pressure. Depending on the type of resectoscope used, the fluid may be a solution containing glycine, sorbitol/mannitol or, more recently, saline. Saline conducts electricity so can only be used with the latest bipolar resectoscopes. Irrigation flushes away blood and tissue trimmings *(see page 144)*, allowing some to be collected for examination under a microscope. Histology reveals a hidden tumor in around 5% of cases.

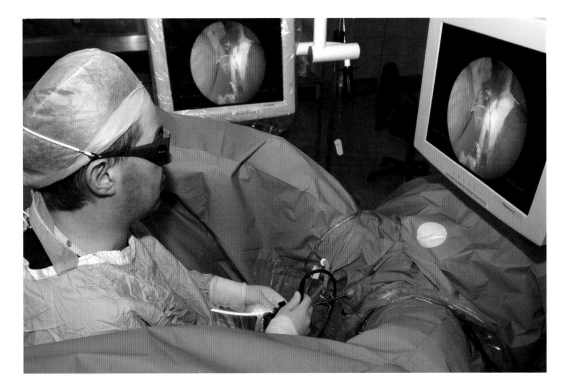

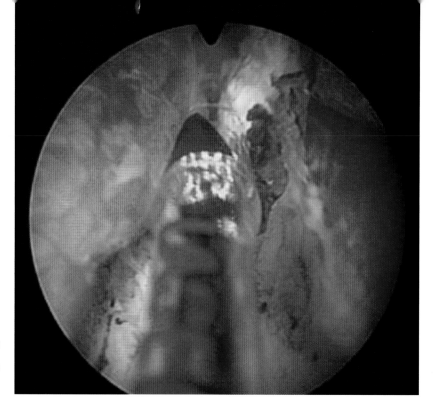

RIGHT An endoscope vision of a laser (yellow) vaporizing prostate tissue within the urethra of a patient with BPH. Debris (brown) is flushed away with saline solution (salt water).

5 The surgeon attempts to remove as much of the enlarged prostate tissue as possible to reduce the chance of post-operative bleeding, infection, and recurrence of BPH. Bleeding points are carefully cauterized to maintain good visualization of tissues. The surgeon may insert a finger in the rectum to push the prostate upward to cut certain parts of the prostate gland more easily.

6 The surgeon tries to finish the procedure within 60 minutes to minimize the amount of irrigation fluid the patient absorbs. Before finishing, he or she carefully inspects the verumontanum, bladder, and surgical field and removes any pieces of resected tissue or hanging tissue tags. Once he or she is satisfied that bleeding has stopped, the endoscope is removed and a catheter inserted into the bladder. A special suppository containing belladonna and opium may be inserted in the rectum to reduce pain and spasm as anesthesia wears off.

Acute retention of urine

One of the most distressing complications of BPH is acute retention of urine. This occurs when the prostate enlarges enough to squeeze the urethra fully closed, so urine cannot leave the bladder. Acute retention of urine is often triggered by spasm of the bladder or pelvic muscles and is made worse by anxiety about not being able to pass water. As urine builds up in the bladder, stretch pains become unbearable and medical help is needed to drain the urine and bring instant relief. This is usually achieved by passing a catheter (flexible tube) into the bladder, through the penis, using a local anesthetic gel to numb the sensitive urethra. Occasionally, if a catheter cannot be passed through the blockage, and the urethra cannot be dilated using special rods, a suprapubic catheter is passed into the expanded bladder through the abdominal wall.

The International Prostate Symptoms Score

The IPSS helps to grade the severity of your prostate symptoms and their impact on your quality of life. There are seven questions with a possible total score of 0–35:

Over the past month, how often have you:	Not at all	<One time in five	< Half the time	Half the time	> Half the time	Almost always
1 Had a sensation of not emptying your bladder completely after you finished urination?	0	1	2	3	4	5
2 Had the urge to urinate again less than two hours after you finished urinating?	0	1	2	3	4	5
3 Found you stopped and started again several times when you urinated?	0	1	2	3	4	5
4 Found it difficult to postpone urination?	0	1	2	3	4	5
5 Had a weak urinary stream?	0	1	2	3	4	5
6 Had to push or strain to begin urination?	0	1	2	3	4	5
Over the past month how many times did you:	**None**	**Once**	**Twice**	**Three times**	**Four times**	**Five or more times**
7 Most typically get up to urinate from the time you went to bed at night until the time you got up in the morning?	0	1	2	3	4	5

In addition, you may be asked a quality of life question to see how you would feel if you were to spend the rest of your life with your urinary condition just the way it is now: Delighted, pleased, mostly satisfied, mixed, mostly dissatisfied, unhappy, or terrible.

Your prostate symptom score, together with the findings of digital rectal examination and PSA level, help your doctor plan your management.

For example:

If you score less than eight, your symptoms are classed as mild and "watchful waiting" may be acceptable to see you how progress.

If you score eight to 19, your symptoms are classed as moderate and medical treatment with drugs may be suggested, assuming the diagnosis of BPH is confirmed.

If you score 20 to 35, your symptoms are classed as severe and surgery may be indicated.

TURP
QUESTIONS & ANSWERS

What are the benefits?

Men who undergo TURP report their BPH symptoms are improved by 80% to 90% at one year after surgery, and are still 60% to 75% improved after five years.

What are the risks?

As well as the general risks associated with surgery and general anesthesia *(see pages 10–11)*, there is an immediate risk of bleeding, and of absorbing excess irrigation fluid during surgery *(see below)*. Long-term complications include urinary incontinence (2% to 3%) and scar tissue formation that interferes with urinary outflow (urethral stricture 2% to 20%).

Are there any alternatives?

Drugs known as 5-a-reductase inhibitors can shrink the prostate gland by blocking an enzyme that converts testosterone to dihydrotestosterone. Other drugs, known as a-blockers (e.g. doxazosin, tamsulosin), relax muscle cells in the prostate gland to reduce spasm. Combination therapy using both an a-blocker and a 5-a-reductase inhibitor can reduce the progression of BPH more than either treatment alone. A natural herbal remedy, saw palmetto, may also help.

Other surgical procedures are available such as radiofrequency ablation, transurethral microwave thermotherapy (TUMT), transurethral needle ablation (TUNA), interstitial laser coagulation (ILC), transurethral vaporization of the prostate (TUVP), and photoselective vaporization of the prostate (PVP) with a "greenlight" laser. Some can be performed as an outpatient procedure. Other surgical approaches include inserting a tubular metal mesh (urethral stent) and balloon dilation of the prostatic urethra. Occasionally open prostatectomy is performed to remove a very enlarged prostate gland through an incision over the pubic bone *(see page 148)*.

What can I do to prepare?

Your doctor may suggest taking a 5-a-reductase inhibitor drug for several weeks before surgery to shrink the gland and minimize bleeding. Try to be as fit and healthy as possible before surgery.

TUR syndrome

Some of the fluid used for continuous irrigation of the urethra is absorbed through cut tissues. Excessive uptake of fluid can cause temporary low sodium levels, blood pressure problems, and confusion. Known as TUR syndrome, it affects around one in 50 men undergoing TURP. Spinal or epidural anesthesia allows the anesthesiologist/surgeon to talk to you and assess your ability to think straight during surgery for early recognition of the problem. Using low fluid pressure reduces the risk.

Stopping smoking can reduce the risk of TUR syndrome, blood clots and infection.

What if I don't have the operation?

If left untreated, BPH can lead to bladder infection (cystitis) due to stagnation of urine trapped in the bladder, the formation of bladder stones due to salts precipitating out of stagnant urine, a total inability to pass water (acute urinary retention) due to complete blocking off the urethra, and kidney damage due to back pressure and back flow of trapped urine.

What happens during the recovery period?

You will have a catheter in the bladder which will drain bright red, blood-stained urine. You may be encouraged to drink plenty of fluids to help flush the catheter through. Bladder spasms and discomfort can be reduced with drugs. After a few days, when swelling has settled, the catheter is removed. At this stage, urine is usually still pink, and urination may sting. It may take up to eight weeks for urinary symptoms to settle. Up to 20% of men experience post-operative problems with intermittent, dribbling incontinence of urine which lasts for several days. In about 5% of cases, this problem is continuous. Pelvic floor exercises can help. You can usually return to work and other normal activities, including sex, within four to six weeks, but avoid strenuous activity and heavy lifting. The prostate usually continues to enlarge so symptoms can recur. Approximately 15% of men require further surgery within eight years.

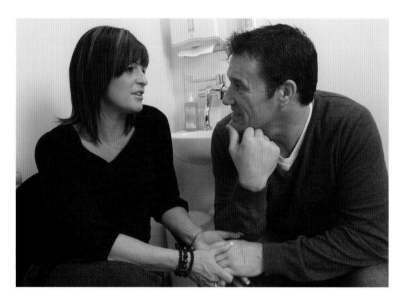

LEFT Possible difficulties with sexual relationships after surgery are one of the unwelcome potential side effects of a TURP.

Sexuality

Some men experience sexual problems after a TURP, with around half noticing a change in the intensity of orgasm. Between 5% and 30% of men experience erectile difficulties after surgery, but this often settles. TURP itself does not seem to increase the risk of long-term erectile dysfunction if this was normal beforehand. Between 30% and 90% of men also develop retrograde ejaculation after prostate surgery, so that sperm pass backward into the bladder during ejaculation. This is not harmful and sperm are passed along with urine next time the bladder is emptied. The condition does cause infertility, however, and medical assistance is needed if you wish to father a child in the future.

OPEN PROSTATECTOMY

Open radical prostatectomy is an operation that removes the prostate gland and two other male glands, the seminal vesicles, through an incision in the lower abdomen. Radical prostatectomy is carried out as part of the treatment for prostate cancer.

WHAT IS THE PROSTATE GLAND?

The prostate is a gland that lies just beneath a man's bladder, wrapped around the urethra — the tube through which urine flows from the bladder to the outside world. It is made up of three parts, a middle (median) lobe and two side (lateral) lobes. The prostate gland secretes a thin, milky fluid that helps to keep the lining of the urethra moist, as well as nourishing sperm. Prostate fluids make up around a third of semen volume. Two other male glands, the seminal vesicles, are attached to the top of the prostate gland. These form coiled, blind sacs that are about 2 in (5 cm) long. They secrete a pale yellow fluid that is rich in fructose sugar, to nourish sperm, plus proteins that allow semen to clot.

PROSTATE CANCER

Prostate cancer is the most common solid tumor to affect adult males. An estimated one in six men over the age of 50 is diagnosed at some time during his life. Although this risk is high, many cancers are picked up early as a result of screening, so that mortality is lower than might otherwise be expected.

Digital rectal examination

The National Cancer Institute recommends that all men over 40 have a digital rectal examination (DRE) once a year to screen for prostate cancer. DRE is important to assess the size, shape, and texture of your prostate gland. The doctor gently inserts a gloved and lubricated finger through your anus into your back passage. Normally, the prostate is smooth and firm, is 0.8 in to 1 in (2 to 3 cm) across, and feels rubbery. Usually, two lobes can be identified, separated by an obvious groove running down the center of the gland. A DRE can confirm whether or not the prostate is enlarged and whether it is tender. It can sometimes also reveal an obvious prostate cancer if the area in reach of the finger feels hard, craggy, irregular, or is tethered to overlying soft tissues. In 90% of cases, prostate cancer arises in the outer parts of the gland where it is often felt as a small, hard lump or irregularity during DRE. If your doctor does find a lump, try not to panic. In half of all cases, no cancer is found — the lump is due to a stone or other benign enlargement. Even if cancer is present, DRE is likely to have caught it early enough in its growth for a good chance of a cure.

OPEN PROSTATECTOMY AT A GLANCE

- **Can it be done as an outpatient?** No. Admission to hospital is necessary.

- **Do I need a general anesthetic?** Laparoscopic procedures usually require general anesthesia. It may be possible to perform an open operation under combined spinal and epidural anesthesia *(see page 8)*.

- **What special tests are needed?** Urine and blood tests check for anemia, infection, and kidney function. Blood levels of the enzyme prostate specific antigen (PSA) are measured. Transrectal ultrasonography of the prostate gland, using a rectal probe inserted through the anus, can reveal the size of a prostate nodule and whether it is solid or cystic (filled with fluid). Transrectal needle biopsy under ultrasound guidance *(see images on pages 150 and 151)* can biopsy suspicious nodules for further examination. The removal of fine cores of prostatic tissue is relatively painless using new biopsy guns.

Computed tomography or MRI scans play a limited role in determining the extent of a tumor. Nuclear isotope bone scans may be performed if PSA is high and bone secondaries are suspected. An alternative is monoclonal antibody technology which can identify prostate tissue spread to other parts of the body.

- **How long does the surgery take?** Open prostatectomy takes between two to three hours.

- **What is the mortality rate?** Around 1 in 1000 (0.1%).

- **How long will I be in hospital?** Patients usually stay in hospital for an average of two to three days.

- **How expensive is it?** 💲💲

- **How many are performed in the US each year?** Around 73,000 open prostatectomy operations are performed in the US each year.

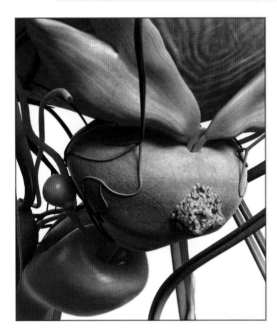

ABOVE Diagram of a prostate cancer on the posterior wall of the prostate gland.

The majority of prostate cancers arise in the outer parts of the prostate gland *(see left)* and tend not to obstruct urinary flow unless the tumor reaches a considerable size. It is therefore difficult to diagnose in the early stages. If obstructive symptoms do occur, they are similar to those of BPH *(see page 140)* but tend to progress more rapidly, over weeks rather than months. Having to get up at night to pass water (nocturia) and passing blood in the urine (hematuria) are also more likely. In the later stages of the disease, non-specific symptoms of cancer may occur, such as tiredness, weight loss, anemia, swollen glands, and pain.

Although most men with prostate cancer do not have a family history of the disease, prostate cancer can have a genetic link. One study found that men with a first-degree relative (father or brother) affected were twice as likely to develop prostate cancer compared to men with no relatives affected. If a second degree relative (uncle, grandfather) had prostate cancer as well, a man's risk increased to eight times that of a male with no affected relatives. Men with either two or three first degree relatives affected had a five- and 11-fold increased risk of developing prostate cancer respectively.

Occasionally an open prostatectomy is needed to treat benign prostate disease if the prostate is very enlarged.

OPEN PROSTATECTOMY
STEP-BY-STEP

NERVE-SPARING TECHNIQUES

A new way to remove the prostate gland, through the abdomen, was developed in the early 1980s. Known as a nerve-sparing radical prostatectomy, this approach helps to preserve the bundle of nerves and blood vessels on either side of the prostate gland that are needed for penile erection. The risk of developing erectile difficulties as a result of surgery is therefore lower than with previous techniques, meaning that more men are now prepared to have their prostate gland removed surgically to treat prostate cancer. This procedure is suitable for men with early prostate cancer that has not spread to surrounding tissues. It is not always possible, however, as the nerves run toward the back of the prostate, which is the most likely place for prostate cancer to spread.

Most open prostatectomy operations are carried out through the abdomen to access the area behind the pubic bone. This is known as an open radical retroperitoneal prostatectomy.

❶ The operating table is tilted head down, so the intestines fall away from the pelvis. The surgeon makes a vertical *(see opposite below)* or horizontal cut along the lower abdomen. The surgeon then carefully cuts through the underlying layers of fat and connective tissue in the abdominal wall, and separates or cuts the muscles to expose the peritoneal membrane that lines the abdominal and pelvic cavities. Rather than cutting through this, however, he tunnels in front of it to remove the fat behind the pubic bone. This is known as an extraperitoneal approach.

RIGHT A surgeon holding a transrectal ultrasound (TRUS) probe with a lubricated sheath. This is inserted into the rectum to monitor the position of needles during prostate biopsy.

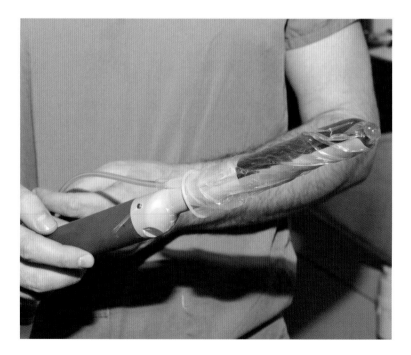

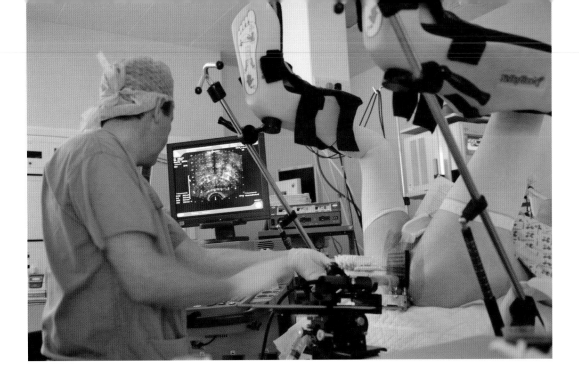

ABOVE A surgeon inserts prostate biopsy needles through the patient's perineum. They are guided to the prostate gland using a transrectal ultrasound probe *(see opposite)*.

❷ Lymph nodes in the area are removed on both sides and sent for examination under a microscope to look for evidence of cancer spread. Pelvic floor muscle fibers and fatty tissue are swept out of the way to expose the front of the prostate gland.

❸ The surgeon carefully excavates the tissues on either side of the prostate gland (using his index fingers) to identify and preserve the nerve bundles which are needed to control erections. The urethra (urinary tube) passing out through the base of the prostate gland is then cut.

RIGHT A surgeon makes the first incision in an open radical prostatectomy operation.

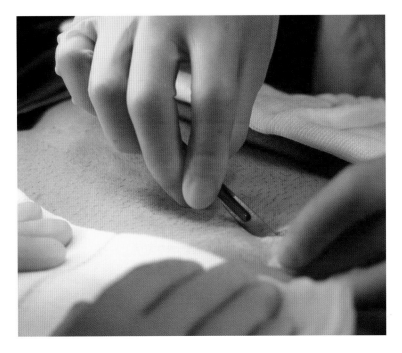

❹ The surgeon pulls the prostate gland upward and uses small clips to close blood vessels (heat sealing is avoided as this might damage the nerve bundles) *(see opposite above)*. The prostate gland and seminal vesicles are carefully separated away from the bladder and rectum, and the two vas deferens (the tubes carrying sperm up from the testicles) are cut and tied.

❺ The urethra between the prostate and bladder is then cut, and the prostate gland and seminal vesicles removed. Tissue is sent for rapid analysis in the laboratory to ensure the edges of surgery are clear of cancer invasion. If cancer cells are found at the surgical edges, more extensive surgery is needed to remove as much cancer tissue as possible. This may have to include the nerve bundles on one or both sides. The surgeon then sews together the two cut ends of the urethra (above and below where the prostate was situated). The connection is checked for leaks by irrigating the bladder with fluid. A urinary catheter is inserted, which will be removed after five days.

❻ The abdominal wound is then closed either with absorbable sutures, that dissolve, or with staples that are removed between three to five days later.

Minimally invasive radical prostatectomy

The prostate gland can be removed using "keyhole" surgery. This may involve the use of robotic arms to move the instruments, controlled by a surgeon sitting at a console. Between four and six small punctures are made in the lower abdomen through which the viewing device (laparoscope) and surgical instruments are inserted.

Some surgeons enter the peritoneal cavity (transperitoneal approach) but it is also possible to operate without puncturing the peritoneal membrane (extraperitoneal approach). In this case, the peritoneal membrane is separated from the abdominal wall, either by pumping in air or by using instruments, fingers, or by inserting an inflatable balloon. The surgeon tunnels down in front of the bladder to reach the prostate gland. The prostate is dissected out from the bladder and surrounding fatty tissues to identify the upper part of the urethra. This is carefully cut, taking care not to damage the bladder neck. The prostate is then carefully cut away, together with the seminal

vesicles, and the vas deferens are cut and tied. Blood vessels are clipped rather than sealed with heat to avoid damaging the nerve bundles needed to control erections. The urethra below the prostate is then cut, and a specimen retrieval bag is introduced through one of the abdominal incisions to collect and remove the freed prostate gland, with seminal vesicles attached. The cut ends of the urethra, above and below where the prostate was situated, are sewn together. The connection is checked for leaks by irrigating the bladder with fluid. A urinary catheter is inserted and the series of abdominal incisions are closed using stitches or clips.

Minimally invasive radical prostatectomy surgery results in less blood loss than open surgery, less post-operative pain, and quicker recovery. Laparoscopic radical prostatectomy takes significantly longer, however, averaging four and a half hours, but if robotic arms are used, surgery time can take less than three hours.

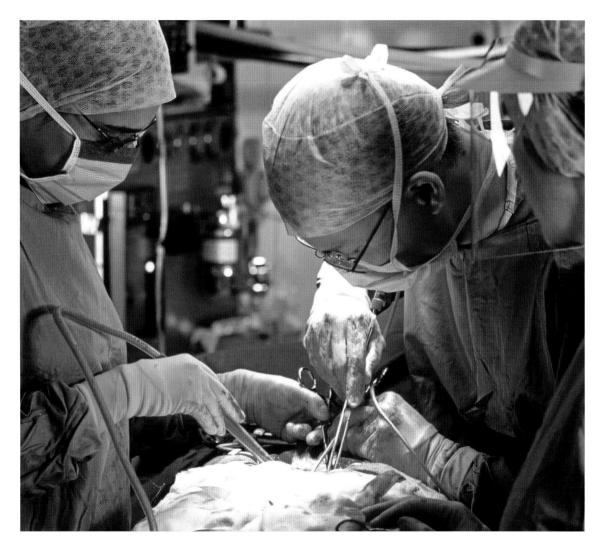

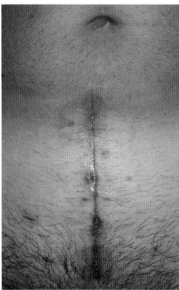

LEFT A scar on the abdomen of a patient, six weeks after he underwent an open radical prostatectomy.

ABOVE Surgeons carefully stopping bleeding during an open radical prostatectomy operation.

Perineal prostatectomy

A less frequent approach is via the perineum — the area found between the scrotum and anus. This is known as a radical perineal prostatectomy. The patient lies on his back with his legs strapped up in stirrups. A curved incision is made behind the scrotum, and the prostate and seminal vesicles are carefully separated away from the rectum and bladder. The cut ends of the urethra are then rejoined and a urinary catheter inserted. This approach is less popular because it does not allow the surgeon to biopsy the lymph nodes in the pubic area. It is also not suitable for removing a very large prostate gland.

OPEN PROSTATECTOMY
QUESTIONS & ANSWERS

What are the benefits?

In early prostate cancer which has not spread, surgery can offer a cure. A study comparing radical prostatectomy to conservative management found that surgery decreased the risk of distant spread (metastasis) and increased survival rates by around 40% over a ten year period.

What are the risks?

As well as the general risks associated with surgery and general anesthesia *(see pages 10–11)*, there is a risk of developing erectile dysfunction (impotence) or urinary incontinence. After nerve-sparing radical prostatectomy between 50% and 70% of men who were previously potent can achieve sexual intercourse, and 10% to 20% may have some urinary incontinence requiring the use of incontinence pads. Results are improved with robotically assisted laparoscopic radical prostatectomy, after which over 80% of men may retain sexual potency. Drugs such as sildenafil can help you to achieve an erection if at least one of the nerve bundles was left intact.

Are there any alternatives?

Radiation therapy can be given as external beam radiotherapy, permanent implantation of radioactive seeds (interstitial brachytherapy), or temporary implantation of a high dose radiation source. The growth of more advanced prostate cancers may be slowed by changing its hormone environment using synthetic hormones (LHRH agonists) that block testosterone production. Occasionally, a surgeon may recommend surgical removal of the testicles (orchidectomy), in which case they can be replaced with egg-shaped implants for an excellent cosmetic result. Unfortunately, chemotherapy with anti-cancer drugs is generally unhelpful.

What can I do to prepare?

Try to be as fit and healthy as possible before surgery, and follow a prostate-friendly diet *(see below)*. Stopping smoking can reduce the risk of blood clots and infection. You may be kept on a liquid diet the day before surgery, and given an enema or laxative to empty your bowel before surgery.

Prostate-friendly diet

Prostate cancer is strongly linked with diet. A high-fat diet, especially animal fat, can double the risk. Consuming a low-fat, high-fiber diet containing good amounts of selenium (e.g. Brazil nuts), lycopene (e.g. cooked tomatoes), vitamin D (e.g. oily fish), and antioxidants (e.g. fruit, vegetables, green tea) may help to reduce the risk of a recurrence. A Japanese style diet containing weak plant hormones (phytoestrogens) also seems to be protective.

What if I don't have the operation?

In the case of small, slow-growing prostate cancers, no treatment may be necessary except regular monitoring; this approach is known as "active surveillance."

What happens during the recovery period?

You may receive pain relief via a patient controlled analgesia pump, as injections into an intravenous drip, or via an epidural. The urinary catheter may be flushed through regularly to prevent it becoming blocked with blood clots. The catheter may be left in place for one to three weeks, and is attached to a bag that will be strapped to your thigh under your trousers *(see left)*. You may experience difficulty passing urine when the catheter is removed, in which case it may be replaced. Stitches or clips are removed after seven to 14 days.

PSA levels are measured regularly, typically every three months for the first two years. If undetectable, they are then measured every six months until five years after surgery, then annually. If PSA levels start to rise, investigations are carried out to look for a local recurrence, or for distant spread.

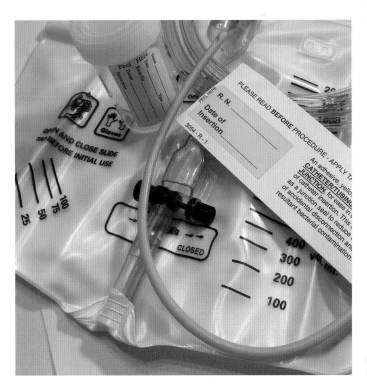

LEFT Sterile flexible catheter and bag used to drain urine from the bladder.

PSA testing

Prostate specific antigen (PSA) is an enzyme produced by prostate cells. It helps to liquefy semen by breaking down the clotted proteins produced by the seminal vesicles. A number of factors can raise the PSA level, including benign prostatic hyperplasia *(see page 141)*, recent ejaculation, and the presence of prostate cancer. It is a more sensitive indicator of prostate cancer than digital rectal examination (DRE) or transrectal ultrasound (TRUS). Unfortunately, the interpretation of PSA levels is not straightforward. One in five men with prostate cancer has normal PSA levels, and one in four men without prostate cancer has raised levels. However, PSA testing plus DRE can increase the detection of cancer by around a third more than DRE alone. A refinement of the test assesses the level of "free" PSA in the blood, which is not bound to protein. The ratio of free PSA to total PSA may be decreased if prostate cancer is present. The use of serial measurements of PSA is also more helpful than a single PSA measurement. Annual screening, together with DRE, is recommended for Caucasian men from the age of 50, and for African American men from the age of 45.

THYROIDECTOMY

A thyroidectomy removes varying amounts of thyroid tissue. It is carried out as part of the treatment for an overactive thyroid gland (hyperthyroidism), to remove an enlarged gland (goiter), or to treat thyroid cancer.

A partial thyroidectomy removes part of the gland, such as one lobe (lobectomy), a total thyroidectomy attempts to remove all visible thyroid tissue, while a subtotal thyroidectomy leaves behind a few grams, near the trachea, to avoid damaging the parathyroid glands *(see page 159)*.

WHAT IS THE THYROID GLAND?

The thyroid is a butterfly-shaped gland at the base of the neck in front of the trachea (windpipe). It has a right and left lobe, joined by a bridge of tissue called the isthmus. In some people, there is an additional remnant of tissue, the pyramidal process, at the top of the gland. The thyroid secretes two iodine-containing hormones, thyroxine (T4) and tri-iodothyronine (T3), which boost metabolism by increasing the speed at which cells work. An under- or over-active thyroid gland therefore affects every part of your body. The thyroid also produces another hormone, calcitonin, which lowers blood calcium levels when they rise above normal.

Thyroid symptoms

The symptoms of an overactive thyroid gland (hyperthyroidism) result from a metabolic rate that is set too high. These include:
- Weight loss, increased appetite.
- Anxiety, irritability, restlessness.
- Tiredness, weakness.
- Rapid pulse, palpitations.
- Sensitivity to heat.
- Diarrhea, menstrual changes.

The symptoms of an underactive thyroid gland (hypothyroidism) are due to a metabolism that is set too slow, including:
- Lack of energy, general slowing down.
- Muscle cramps and weakness.
- Increasing weight.
- Feeling the cold.
- Dry skin, brittle hair, loss of outer third of eyebrows.
- Thickening of tissues in the face and limbs.
- Slow pulse.
- Constipation, heavy periods.
- A deepening voice which may seem slurred.

THYROIDECTOMY AT A GLANCE

- **Can it be done as an outpatient?** No. Admission to hospital is necessary.

- **Do I need a general anesthetic?** Usually, yes. Occasionally thyroidectomy is performed under local anesthesia but this is unusual.

- **What special tests are needed?** Thyroid function is assessed by measuring blood levels of thyroid stimulating hormone (TSH, made in the pituitary gland) and thyroxine hormone (T4). Most T4 is bound to protein and inactive, so only free (unbound) thyroxine is measured (FT4). A high FT4 and low TSH suggests an overactive thyroid gland (hyperthyroidism). A low FT4 and high TSH suggests an underactive thyroid gland (hypothyroidism). Levels of tri-iodothyronine (T3) are not usually measured in their own right but may be used to calculate free thyroxine levels more accurately (free thyroxine index). Blood tests to look for antithyroid antibodies are performed if an autoimmune inflammation of the gland (thyroiditis) is suspected.

  If a thyroid nodule is present, cells may be collected for examination under a microscope. Known as fine needle aspiration biopsy, cells are sucked out using a tiny hypodermic needle and syringe, often under ultrasound guidance. This is repeated two or three times in different parts of the nodule. Local anesthetic is not usually needed.

  Thyroid imaging to assess the volume of the gland, and the hormone-secreting activity of nodules may be performed using radionuclide scanning (with technetium or radioactive iodine) or ultrasound. Computed tomography (CT) or magnetic resonance imaging (MRI) help to assess thyroid tissues (e.g. goiter) that have grown down behind the sternum.

- **How long does the surgery take?** One to two hours.

- **What is the mortality rate?** One in 500 (0.2%).

- **How long will I be in hospital?** Patients usually stay in hospital for an average of two days.

- **How expensive is it?** 💲

- **How many are performed in the US each year?** Around 57,000 operations are performed to remove all or part of the thyroid gland each year. Thyroid conditions are more common in women, and four times more females require thyroidectomy than males.

WHEN IS IT NECESSARY?

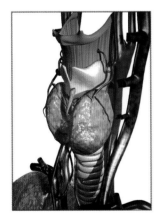

ABOVE Illustration of a cancerous nodule on the thyroid gland.

Partial thyroidectomy is sometimes needed to treat an overactive thyroid gland (hyperthyroidism). It may be recommended when medical approaches such as antithyroid drugs (e.g. propylthiouracil, methimazole) or radioactive iodine (which concentrates in the thyroid to deactivate thyroid cells) have not worked, or are contraindicated (for example, radioactive iodine is not suitable during pregnancy).

Subtotal or total thyroidectomy may be suggested to treat a large goiter (swollen thyroid gland) especially if multiple nodules are present, if the gland is pressing on structures such as the windpipe to restrict breathing, or if the swelling is unsightly.

It may also be necessary when a single lump (nodule) forms within the gland. Removal of a single thyroid nodule is advisable if it is large (1.2 in / 3 cm across or more), or if cancer is suspected. Thyroid cancer in a single nodule may be treated by removing the lobe containing the nodule, together with the central part (isthmus) of the thyroid gland or, more usually, with a total thyroidectomy. The procedure selected depends on your age, type, and extent of cancer.

Thyroidectomy
Step-by-step

Open thyroidectomy

Before having an operation on the thyroid gland, it is important to ensure thyroid function is as normal as possible, either by taking medication to damp down over-secretion of thyroid hormones, or to replenish levels if hypothyroidism is present. The risks of surgery increase where a patient has very abnormal thyroid function.

The majority of single thyroid nodules are benign (non-cancerous), but all are investigated to determine their nature, usually with a fine needle aspiration biopsy. The results are classified as benign, malignant (cancerous), or indeterminate. As around one in four of those classed as indeterminate are later found to contain cancer, the surgeon may either proceed straight to surgery, or request a radioiodine scintigraphy scan to help plan whether a partial or total thyroidectomy is needed.

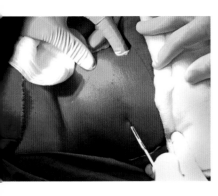

ABOVE Starting the incision at the bottom of the neck.

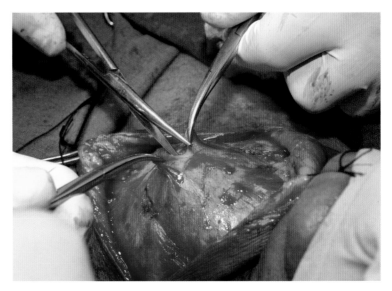

RIGHT A combination of sharp and blunt dissection is used to separate the tissues over the thyroid gland.

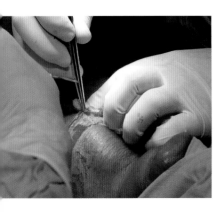

ABOVE A patient undergoing a thyroid lobectomy.

The scan involves taking a low dose of radioactive iodine as a liquid or capsule. This is taken up by the thyroid gland and a scan is performed to see how much iodine enters the nodule compared with the remaining thyroid tissue. A nodule that takes up less iodine is described as "cold," one that takes up a similar amount to surrounding tissues is "warm," and one that actively concentrates more iodine is classed as "hot." Cancer-containing nodules are usually "cold" (although most cold nodules are not cancerous).

A warm nodule is usually benign. A "hot" toxic nodule, associated with hyperthyroidism, will need medical treatment with antithyroid drugs before partial thyroidectomy. The thyroid scan may also show up multiple nodules when only one was previously seen or felt — even the best surgeon is unlikely to detect a nodule that is less than 0.4 in (1 cm) across.

❶ Having decided whether to perform a partial, subtotal, or total thyroidectomy, the surgeon makes a horizontal incision, about 3 in (8 cm) long, at the base of the neck *(see opposite top)*. The incision is made within a normal skin crease, where your skin folds as you bend your head forward, to help minimize the appearance of the scar. If the surgeon plans to remove lymph nodes as part of the treatment for thyroid cancer, the incision turns up toward the ear at one or both ends.

❷ The surgeon cuts through the fat beneath the skin, and a thin layer of muscle called the platysma *(see opposite center and below)*. The edges of the incision are then pulled open, and the underlying strap-like muscles retracted to either side to reveal the thyroid gland.

❸ The surgeon carefully frees the thyroid gland from the trachea (windpipe) and larynx (voicebox) to which it is firmly attached. The two superior thyroid arteries, which enter the thyroid from above, and

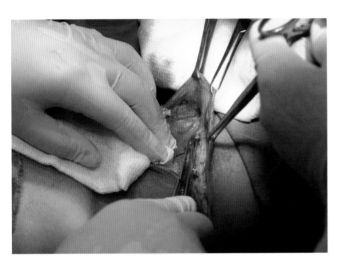

BELOW Careful dissection is needed to minimize bleeding.

the two inferior thyroid arteries entering the thyroid from below are identified. The surgeon also looks for a fifth artery, which is sometimes present, leading into the central part of the gland. If performing a total thyroidectomy, all these arteries are tied off and cut, along with thyroid veins at the top and sides. If carrying out a partial or subtotal thyroidectomy, the surgeon ties off and cuts only those vessels supplying the part of the thyroid to be removed. In this case, he or she usually also removes the small pyramidal lobe (if present) at the top of the gland; otherwise this might later enlarge to cause a visible swelling at the front of the neck.

❹ The surgeon carefully identifies and preserves the parathyroid glands behind the thyroid, and the two recurrent laryngeal nerves.

Parathyroid glands

The parathyroid glands are situated behind the thyroid, at the top and bottom of each lobe, sharing its blood supply. Their positions and number are variable. Although most people have four, some people have three, five, or six parathyroid glands. These small structures secrete parathyroid hormone (or parathormone) which raises calcium levels when they fall below normal (the opposite action to thyroid calcitonin hormone). With a total thyroidectomy, preserving the parathyroid glands is not always possible. In this case, one or two glands are inserted into a muscle in the neck, shoulder, or non-dominant forearm, where they usually survive and function well. Early post-operative signs of low calcium levels (hypocalcemia) include numbness and pins and needles around the mouth, and spasm of facial muscles when the cheek is tapped over the facial nerve. If necessary, calcium is given orally or intravenously.

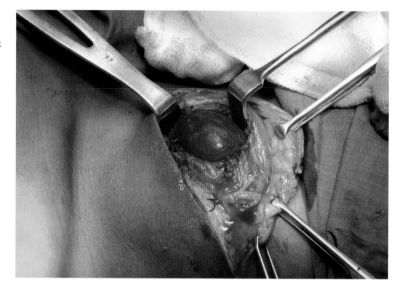

RIGHT A thyroid cyst is exposed as the strap muscles of the neck are pulled to the sides with small retractors.

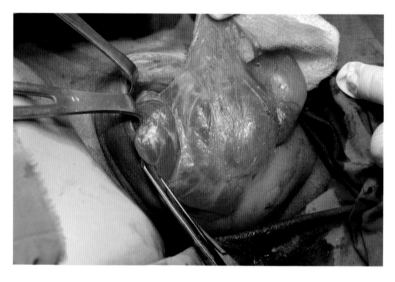

❺ For thyroidectomy to treat cancer, lymph nodes in the center of the neck are removed. Other nodes in the side of the neck are assessed and may be sent for immediate analysis to look for cancer cells. If present, these lymph nodes are carefully removed in a modified radical neck dissection.

❻ If a lot of tissue is removed, a drain may be inserted for a day or two to prevent a build-up of fluid, but this is usually unnecessary.

ABOVE Exposing the thyroid gland in this patient reveals multiple cysts.

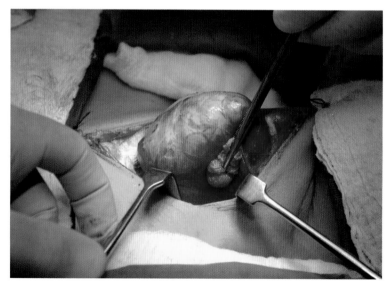

RIGHT The surgeon swabs away blood while looking for the middle thyroid vein.

The recurrent laryngeal nerves

The recurrent laryngeal nerves, which run on either side of the thyroid gland, control movement of the vocal cords. Surgeons take care to preserve these nerves where possible, but they may have to be sacrificed if involved within a cancerous growth. In the case of a small thyroid cancer, less than 0.6 in (1.5 cm) in diameter, some surgeons may recommend leaving behind a tiny amount of thyroid tissue (less than 0.035 oz / one gram) to guarantee preservation of at least one recurrent laryngeal nerve. Other surgeons always perform a total thyroidectomy as post-operative scanning for evidence of new tumors is easier when no normal thyroid tissue remains to take up radioactive iodine. Damaging, or removing, one recurrent laryngeal nerve leads to a permanent hoarse voice. Damage or removing both nerves can require tracheotomy (a tube inserted into the front of the windpipe) to ensure you can breathe properly. Permanent accidental damage to these nerves is rare, occurring around once in every 250 operations.

RIGHT **The surgeon ties off vessels with a silk ligature.**

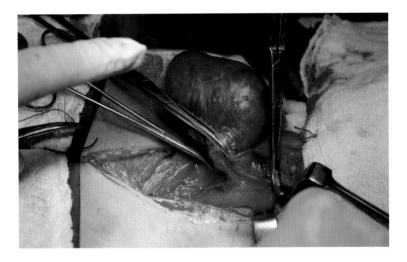

Minimally invasive thyroid surgery

A minimally invasive, video-assisted technique may be used to remove a small thyroid nodule (less than 1.2 in / 3 cm in size) for immediate examination under a microscope. A small horizontal incision is made 0.8 in (2 cm) above the sternum, in the midline, where bleeding is minimal. This is higher than for traditional open surgery. Fat and the platysma muscle are carefully cut through, and deeper strap muscles are moved aside with small retractors. A viewing device (endoscope) is inserted through the incision and the nodule dissected under endoscopic or video-assisted vision, using tiny instruments. Three people are now needed: The surgeon, an assistant to hold the retractors, and an endoscopist to control the endoscope. Blood vessels are clipped, or sealed, then cut. Saline may be injected with a syringe to flush away blood and maintain a clear view. After freeing up the thyroid lobe, taking care to preserve the recurrent laryngeal nerve and parathyroid glands, the surgeon removes the endoscope and retractors. Using forceps, the freed lobe is carefully pulled outside the body, through the incision, and the isthmus is cut under direct vision. If necessary, the other lobe may be removed in the same way, through the same midline incision, to complete a total thyroidectomy. After checking for any bleeding, the platysma muscle and skin are closed with an absorbable suture, and the small skin wound closed with sutures or skin glue. There is minimal scarring, and a quicker return to work following this procedure.

THYROIDECTOMY
QUESTIONS & ANSWERS

What are the benefits?

Thyroidectomy will improve symptoms due to hyperthyroidism or goiter. It offers the chance of a cure for thyroid cancer that has not spread to lymph nodes or distant organs.

What are the risks?

As well as the general risks associated with surgery and general anesthesia *(see pages 10–11)*, the trauma of thyroid surgery can cause the parathyroid glands to stop working temporarily. If not treated, low calcium levels lead to muscle spasm (tetany). The glands usually recover within a few days. In one in 300 cases, they do not recover function and oral vitamin D and calcium supplements are needed for life.

Damage to the recurrent laryngeal nerves *(see page 161)* can cause temporary or permanent hoarseness. The superior laryngeal nerve above the thyroid gland is occasionally damaged, leading to voice fatigue and reduced vocal range.

Are there any alternatives?

A single benign (non-cancerous) nodule may simply be observed, if the diagnosis is certain. A overactive thyroid gland may be treated medically with antithyroid drugs or radioactive iodine (radioablation).

What can I do to prepare?

If you have hyperthyroidism, you usually take antithyroid medication for four to six weeks before surgery. You may also take iodine for ten days before surgery to reduce the size of the thyroid and the blood vessels supplying it. A beta-blocker drug can reduce symptoms such as a rapid heartbeat or trembling. Hypothyroidism is treated with thyroid hormone medication to obtain normal thyroid function.

What if I don't have the operation?

Medical treatment can control an overactive thyroid gland, but surgery may be needed if this fails or is contraindicated. A goiter may continue to grow and restrict breathing if not removed. A thyroid cancer may continue to grow, or spread, if not removed.

What happens during the recovery period?

Calcium levels are checked to ensure the parathyroid glands are working. This is carried out every six to eight hours after a total thyroidectomy.

After total thyroidectomy, thyroid hormone replacement therapy is needed, with T4 or T4 plus T3, depending on your physician's preference. Postoperative scanning is done to look for residual thyroid tissue and radioactive iodine given to ablate any undetected thyroid. With partial thyroidectomy and lobectomy, thyroid function is

Thyroid hormone replacement

Most T3 hormone in your body is formed from the conversion of T4 at sites other than the thyroid gland (e.g. liver, kidneys, pancreas), so you may only receive thyroid replacement therapy in the form of synthetic T4. Some doctors suggest that people with hypothyroidism feel better if they take a mixture of T3 and T4 rather than T4 alone. This treatment is controversial, however, and opinions may change. This is something you may wish to discuss with your doctor if you do not feel as well as you would like, despite taking adequate amounts of T4.

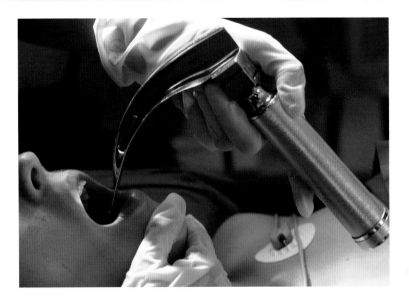

RIGHT An anesthesiologist prepares to insert a laryngoscope.

monitored regularly to see if thyroid hormone replacement should become necessary *(see box above)*.

Recovery from thyroid surgery usually takes one to two weeks, during which your neck feels stiff and tender. You may have a temporary hoarse voice, cough, and pain on swallowing. Direct laryngoscopy (visualization of the vocal cords) may be performed if you experience persistent hoarseness or shortness of breath.

You can return to driving as soon as your head can turn without difficulty. Many people with benign thyroid conditions return to work after two to three weeks.

Depending on how much thyroid tissue was removed, you may need to take thyroid hormone replacement tablets *(see above)*. In the case of thyroid cancer, enough thyroid hormone is given to suppress production of thyroid-stimulating hormone (TSH) in the pituitary gland. This helps to reduce the chance of any remaining thyroid cells regrowing.

If thyroid cancer is diagnosed, a scan (radioiodine scintigraphy) may be carried out six weeks after surgery to look for spread of thyroid cancer cells, particularly in the lungs.

You may be advised to take iodine supplements if you had a goiter linked with iodine deficiency, or if you were exposed to radioactive iodine as part of your work-up or treatment.

SKIN GRAFTING

Skin grafting is a technique in which a thin layer of skin is completely detached from a donor area and used to cover a new area where skin is missing. The skin defect may result from congenital abnormalities, trauma, burns, surgical reconstruction, or the surgical treatment of cancer. Skin may also be removed because it is diseased, scarred, or features an unwanted mole, birthmark, or tattoo.

WHAT IS SKIN?

Skin is the largest organ in the body. It forms a waterproof barrier against the outside world, protecting against physical damage, dehydration, and infection. Skin has two main layers, an outer epidermis and an inner dermis, each of which is several cell thicknesses deep. The epidermis makes up around 5% of the total skin thickness, and the dermis accounts for the remaining 95%. The lowest level of the epidermis, the basal layer, continually divides to produce new cells which push up toward the surface. As they move upward, they are filled with a tough protein called keratin. The cells become flattened, hardened, and die to produce an outer protective layer that is continually worn away and replaced.

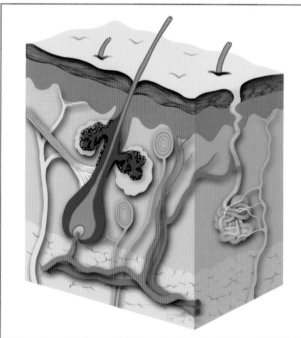

ABOVE An illustration showing a cross section through the skin.

Whereas the epidermis is composed mostly of dead skin cells, the dermis is made up of living cells. It contains collagen and elastin fibers, which give skin its tone and strength, plus blood vessels, nerve endings, sweat glands, sebaceous (oil) glands, and hair follicles.

Because skin is so vital to protect against infection, any defects must be closed as soon as possible. If the area is too large to simply sew together, a skin graft is needed. A skin graft may contain part of the thickness of the skin — known as a split skin graft — or the full thickness of the skin.

SPLIT SKIN GRAFTS

A split skin graft is a sheet of tissue containing epidermis and some dermis. It is harvested from a donor site by shaving the skin with a sharp blade. This leaves behind a layer of deep dermis which, when cared for properly, can become recovered (re-epithelialized) by new skin cells growing in from the sides.

The donor site is carefully chosen, and may include the inner part of the arm or thigh, where the resulting wound will be well hidden. Other popular sites for harvesting skin includes the abdomen, buttocks, or scalp. Thin split skin grafts have the highest chance of "taking," while thick split skin grafts are more durable and give a more acceptable cosmetic result.

FULL THICKNESS SKIN GRAFTS

A full thickness skin graft is a sheet of tissue containing epidermis and the full layer of dermis. This gives an even better cosmetic result than a thick split skin graft, as it tends to contract less. It does, however, need to be applied to a recipient site that has an excellent blood supply.

Full thickness grafts are most commonly used on the face and hands after the removal of a small lesion. They are not used to cover large wounds, however, as their removal leaves a deficit at the donor site that needs to be recovered. They are harvested from areas that are well-hidden (e.g. from behind the ear, or in the groin), or which have surplus skin that is easily sewn together afterward (e.g. above the collar bone, or from upper eyelids that might benefit from a "tuck").

Skin regeneration

Skin can regenerate if the basal layer of the epidermis is intact, or if the area is small enough for new cells to grow in from the sides. If the basal layer is destroyed, however, (for example as a result of a third degree burn) skin grafting is needed to cover the area of tissue loss.

Skin Grafting
Step-by-step

Harvesting healthy skin

A small skin graft, such as that needed to repair small areas of skin loss on the hand or fingers, may be harvested using a local anesthetic. If a large split skin graft is required, however, this is usually obtained under general anesthesia. Both the donor and recipient sites are carefully washed with antiseptic to help reduce the risk of infection.

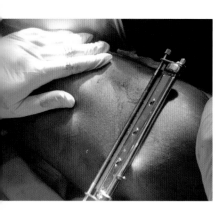

ABOVE Preparing to harvest donor skin.

BELOW A surgeon removes skin from the patient's torso using a sawing motion.

❶ The surgeon marks out the donor area of skin, such as on the inner arm or thigh, taking care to harvest more than enough skin to cover the recipient site (elastin fibers cause some contraction of removed skin). If harvesting a small graft, local anesthetic is injected into the area to numb it. Epinephrine is included in the mix as this causes blood vessels to constrict so that bleeding is reduced. If performing a full thickness graft, the surgeon usually plans to take an ellipse-shaped patch of skin so that the edges of the harvest site can easily be sewn together afterward to close the wound.

❷ The surgeon lubricates the marked area of skin, and the knife blade, with liquid paraffin. If taking a split skin graft, an assistant grips the part of the body, such as the arm or leg, with a sterile swab to tense the skin and form a rounded surface *(see left)*.

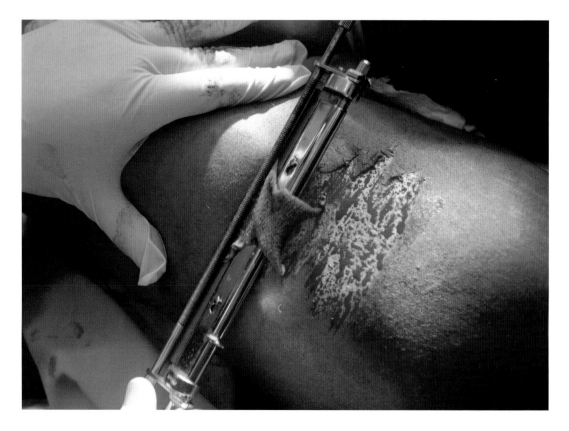

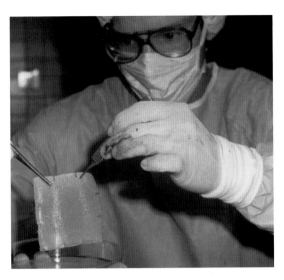

ABOVE A surgeon holding a sheet of cultured human skin.

❸ The surgeon then shaves the split skin graft from the area using a special knife, rather like a carpenter's plane, or an electric blade called a dermatome. The blade can be set to take the appropriate thickness of skin graft, and is advanced a few millimeters at a time, using a sawing action *(see opposite below)*. When taking a large split skin graft, special boards are used to tense the skin on either side of the knife. If taking a full thickness graft, the surgeon uses a scalpel to remove an ellipse of skin, together with some underlying subcutaneous tissue.

❹ The harvested skin graft is placed upside down onto a moist, sterile swab and assessed to see whether it is large enough. If not, another strip is taken. If preparing a full thickness graft, the subcutaneous tissues are cut away using small, curved scissors. Sometimes, a composite graft consisting of skin, subcutaneous fat, plus muscle or cartilage may be used — for example, to repair a nostril or part of the ear.

The donor site may be dressed with special dressings (e.g. calcium alginate), paraffin gauze, dressing gauze, and a crepe bandage. There is increasing use of occlusive, semi-permeable polyurethane dressings that significantly reduce pain and which promote more rapid, moist wound healing.

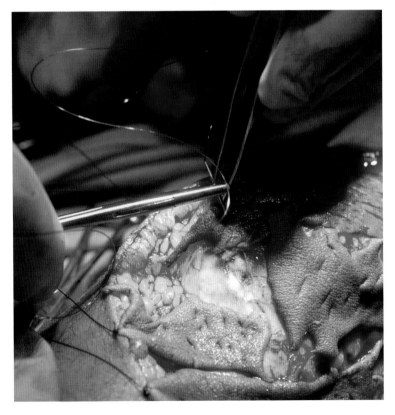

RIGHT Surgeons carefully stitch donor skin during transplantation. The pores in the skin widen to help mold the graft in place.

PLACING THE GRAFT

❺ The recipient site, which will receive the graft, must be properly prepared to maximize the chances of the graft surviving *(see below)*. In some cases, the surgeon creates the recipient site at the same time as preparing the graft, by removing an area of diseased or scarred tissue. In this case, pressure is applied over the wound to stop bleeding before the skin graft is applied. Sterile gauze soaked in an epinephrine solution may be used to constrict blood vessels, too.

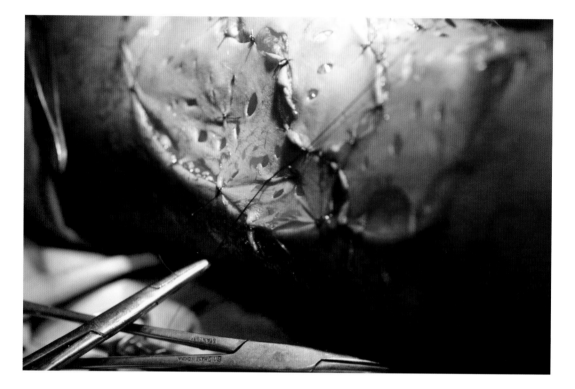

ABOVE **A close-up of a suture being placed in the border of a graft.**

Preparing the recipient site

For optimal survival, the graft needs a clean "bed" with healthy, uninfected underlying tissues that have a good blood supply. Thin split skin grafts therefore survive more readily than thick split skin grafts or full thickness grafts because oxygen and nutrients pass through more easily to nourish the detached cells as they take root and start to grow. If the recipient site is infected, it is treated with antiseptic dressings that are changed three to four times a day, and antibiotics are prescribed. It is only ready for grafting when the infection has cleared and the tissues look healthy. Grafts "take" best on exposed muscle or areas of granulation tissue, which grow up from the underlying connective tissues as part of the healing process. Granulation tissue forms a moist, red, bumpy surface with a good blood supply. Skin grafts do not take well on exposed fat as this has a poor blood supply. Skin grafting is not suitable where there are exposed underlying structures, such as bare tendons, bone, cartilage, large blood vessels, nerves, or intestines.

Maximizing chances of success

Quilted grafts are used when covering highly vascularized areas, such as the tongue, which will bleed and loosen the graft if stitched around the edges as normal. Instead, individual stitches are placed over the whole area of the graft, as with a bed quilt, to assist "taking" at multiple sites.

Meshed grafts are used when the supply of donor skin is insufficient to cover the necessary area (for example, after extensive burns), or to reduce the risk of oozing separating the graft (e.g. on the lower leg). Long, thin strips of split skin graft are harvested and passed through a skin mesher. This cuts a pattern into the skin (rather like when making a lattice pastry pie topping) so it can be stretched and stitched into place to cover a wider area. After grafting, skin cells grow from the lattice to cover the gaps within one week. These grafts are less durable, however, and the mesh pattern remains after healing, making them unsuitable for the face *(see below)*.

Delayed exposed grafting is necessary when it is difficult to stop bleeding at a freshly prepared recipient site. The split skin graft is spread, upside down, onto paraffin gauze, folded, and wrapped in a moist swab. It is stored in sterile conditions in a refrigerator. The graft is applied to the recipient site the next day and left exposed for regular observation. Any serum collecting underneath it is carefully massaged out so the new skin remains in close contact with the underlying flesh.

RIGHT A split thickness skin graft.

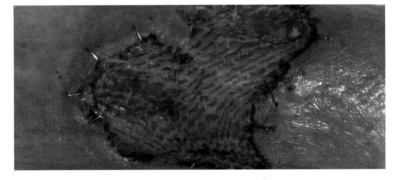

BELOW A bandage is applied over a completed skin graft.

❻ The harvested sheet of skin is applied directly onto the recipient site, cut (opaque) side down, and carefully spread out using non-toothed forceps. Any surplus skin is cut off to leave an overlapping margin of around 0.1 in (3 mm) at the edges. The graft is anchored in place using a few sutures at the edges *(see opposite)*, unless it is in a site where a good compression dressing can be applied.

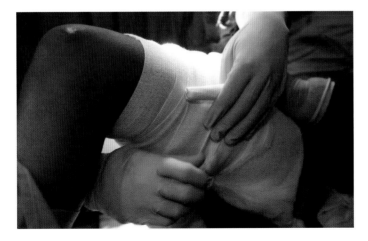

The graft is covered with paraffin gauze, dressing gauze, cotton wool, and adhesive dressings. A compression bandage helps to keep the skin firmly in contact with underlying flesh, and reduces the risk of oozing which could cause it to separate *(see left)*. Negative pressure (vacuum) dressings are also popular.

Skin Grafting
Questions & Answers

What are the benefits?

Grafting covers a vulnerable area that has lost its skin to reduce the risk of infection, and to reduce pain by covering exposed nerve endings. It may also improve the cosmetic appearance of the area.

What are the risks?

As well as the general risks associated with surgery and general anesthesia *(see pages 10–11)*, you may develop infection at the donor or recipient site. Infection at the recipient site means the graft may fail. Infection at the donor site may impair healing. The donor site may develop unsightly scarring or show changes in skin pigmentation or hair development.

Are there any alternatives?

Synthetic skin substitutes are available for temporary wound coverage to help reduce infection and fluid loss. Grafts obtained from cadavers or pigs can also be used as temporary biological dressings to stimulate granulation tissue formation. They are eventually rejected, however, (usually within ten days unless immunosuppressant drugs are taken) and are then removed before proceeding to skin grafting. Skin grafts may be grown in a culture from a patient's own, harvested skin cells. These cultured epidermal autografts (CEAs) only contain epithelial cells and are usually very thin. They have a higher rate of infection and graft loss than normal skin grafts which contain a part of the dermis. Dermal grafts that do not contain any cells, but which act as a scaffold on which cells from underlying tissue can grow through, are available, however. Once these become revascularized, over a period of seven to 21 days, an ultra-thin split thickness graft (or a cultured epidermal autograft) may be placed on top.

What can I do to prepare?

Try to ensure that you are as healthy as possible. Eat a nutritious diet, and maintain a good fluid intake to ensure your tissues are well hydrated. If you smoke, do your utmost to stop. Some surgeons may postpone or even cancel your operation if you are unable to refrain from smoking for at least six weeks before **and** six weeks after surgery, as this reduces the chance of the graft taking. Two weeks before surgery, you may be asked to discontinue taking certain drugs and herbal remedies, especially those that may increase bleeding time.

What if I don't have the operation?

Areas of the body that are not covered with skin will soon become infected.

What happens during the recovery period?

Where possible, a compression dressing is applied for 24 hours to keep the skin graft firmly in contact with underlying tissues. The part of the body with the graft is kept elevated after the operation to reduce oozing that might separate the skin from underlying tissues. If the graft is below your knee, you will not be allowed to put your leg down for a period of seven days.

The donor site is typically more painful than the recipient site, especially during the first 24 to 48 hours, but usually heals within seven days. New blood vessels grow into the lower level of the graft within four to seven days. During this vulnerable time, the graft must be protected from pressure and movement, especially shear forces (for

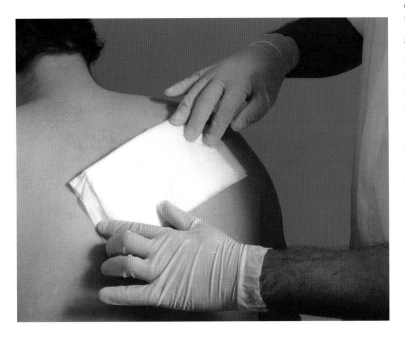

ABOVE The donor site is protected with a dressing after a skin graft has been harvested.

example, when one part of the body, such as the arm, rubs against another part of the body, such as the chest wall). When you start to slowly mobilize, the graft will be protected with compression dressings that keep it firmly in place. Nerve endings grow into the graft two to four weeks after placement, when some feeling may start to return. Hair follicles transplanted from the donor site may grow on a full thickness graft, but a split skin graft remains hairless.

Both the recipient and donor site are disturbed as little as possible, and are typically redressed after one week. The skin graft must be protected from trauma for two to three weeks. Avoid strenuous exercise and lifting. Depending on the site and size of the graft, and your occupation, you may be able to return to work within a few days of surgery. If grafting is extensive, or on your lower leg, however, you may have to stay in hospital or off work for several weeks.

A split skin graft needs regular moisturizing as it does not contain oil or sweat glands.

Let your doctor know if:

- You develop a fever.
- You develop increasing pain, swelling, redness, or warmth at the donor or recipient sites.
- You experience excessive pain that is not helped with medication.
- You develop bleeding or a smelly discharge at the donor or recipient sites.

Glossary

Adenoidectomy Surgical removal of the adenoids commonly performed along with tonsillectomy.

Adenoids Lymph tissue in the back of the throat, above the tonsils.

Adhesions Strands of fibrous tissue that can form within a body cavity following surgery, as part of the healing process.

Anastomosis Surgical joining of two tissues to form a connection e.g. between two cut ends of a blood vessel, or between two cut ends of a loop of bowel.

Angioplasty A surgical procedure in which narrowing of an artery is corrected by the insertion of a narrow, flexible tube (catheter) on the end of which is a balloon. Inflating the balloon at the site of narrowing helps to widen it. A stent may be inserted at the same time.

Appendectomy Surgical removal of the vermiform appendix.

Appendicitis Inflammation of the vermiform appendix.

Artery A type of blood vessel that carries blood away from the heart. All arteries, except for the pulmonary arteries (and the umbilical artery during pregnancy), carry oxygenated blood.

Bile A yellow-green fluid secreted by liver cells (hepatocytes). Bile is stored in the gallbladder and is squirted into the duodenum during digestion to aid the digestion of dietary fats.

Bypass graft The surgical insertion of a new circulation around a blocked artery through which blood can flow. The graft may be artificial or made from a non-essential artery or vein taken from another part of the body.

Carpal tunnel An anatomical space in the wrist between the wrist bones (carpals) and an overlying band of tissue (transverse carpal ligament).

Cataract A cloudy opacity in the eye lens that obscures vision.

Cataract extraction Surgical removal of a clouded eye lens. An artificial lens is normally inserted to correct vision.

Cauterize Using hot instruments to seal tissues and to stop bleeding.

Cesarean section The surgical delivery of a baby through an incision in the mother's abdominal wall and uterus.

Cholangiogram An imaging technique that outlines the bile ducts.

Cholangitis Inflammation of the gallbladder.

Cholecystectomy Surgical removal of the gallbladder (cholecyst).

Coagulation Clotting of blood. Heat (electrocautery) can be used to seal (cauterize) tissues and coagulate vessels to stop bleeding during surgery.

Colic A type of pain that comes and goes in waves. This is typical of the pain experienced when gallstones obstruct the bile ducts

Colorectal resection Surgical removal of part of the large bowel (colon and/or rectum).

Colostomy An artificial connection made between part of the large bowel (colon) and the abdominal wall.

Curette A sharp, spoon-shaped surgical instrument used to cut and scoop out tissues, for example during adenoidectomy.

Drain A drainage tube used to remove body fluids after surgery. This helps to prevent a build-up of infection.

Electrocautery A process in which tissue is destroyed by heat conducted through a metal probe by an electric current.

Endarterectomy A surgical procedure in which an artery is cut open and the lining cleaned of material (atherosclerotic plaque) that is furring it up to cause a narrowing.

Epidural anesthesia A form of local anesthetic in which drugs are injected into the epidural space surrounding the spinal cord.

Forceps A hinged instrument used to grasp and hold tissues during surgery.

Gallstones Solid collections of material that can precipitate out of bile to form stones in the gallbladder.

Graft A surgical procedure to transplant human or artificial tissue into the body.

Harmonic scalpel A surgical blade in which ultrasonic vibration produces heat which is used to cut and seal tissues.

Hernia A bulge produced when an internal part of the body pushes through a weakness in the tissues that normally contain it.

Herniorrhaphy Surgical repair of a hernia.

Hysterectomy Removal of the female uterus (womb).

Ileostomy An artificial connection made between part of the small bowel (ileum) and the abdominal wall.

Incision A surgical cut made to gain access to deeper tissues of the body.

Incisional hernia Protrusion of internal body parts (typically intestines) through a weakness in a surgical scar to cause a bulge at the site of previous surgery.

Inguinal hernia A hernia that pushes through the abdominal wall in the region of the inguinal canal.

Laminectomy Surgical removal of part of a back bone (vertebra).

Laparoscope A viewing device used to look inside the body. There are two types: a telescopic lens system connected to a video camera, and a digital device which uses a fiber optic system.

Laparoscopy A minimally invasive form of surgery. The surgeon operates through one or more small incisions, through which are inserted a viewing device and tiny surgical instruments.

Laparotomy An incision through the abdominal wall to allow exploration of the abdominal organs.

Laser A device that emits light through a process called stimulated emission. Special lasers that emit heat can be used to cut and seal tissues during surgery.

Ligament A strong, fibrous band of tissue that connects bones together within joints. Folds within the membrane lining the abdominal and pelvic cavities are also referred to as ligaments, e.g. the broad ligament that supports the uterus.

Lumpectomy Surgical removal of a lump. This term usually refers to the removal of a breast lump.

Lymph node A small structure that forms part of the lymphatic system. Lymph nodes are found throughout the body and act like filters to trap foreign particles, such as bacteria. They contain immune cells (leucocytes) that help to identify and fight infections. Lymph nodes become enlarged when they are actively fighting an infection or other disease.

Mastectomy The surgical removal of a breast.

Minimally invasive procedure Any procedure that is less invasive than traditional open surgery used to treat the same condition. It typically involves the use of a laparoscope.

Oophorectomy Removal of the female ovaries.

Peritoneum A sheet of tissue (peritoneal membrane) that lines the inner surface of the abdominal and pelvic cavity and the outer surface of the abdominal and pelvic organs.

Phacoemulsification Surgical procedure in which the eye lens is fragmented using ultrasound and removed by sucking it out of the eye through a special needle.

Prostate gland A gland found at the base of the bladder in men.

Prostatectomy Surgical removal of part or all of the prostate gland.

Prosthesis An artificial body part, such as an artificial joint or an artificial eye lens.

Resection The surgical removal of part or all of a body organ or structure.

Retractors Surgical instruments used to spread open skin incisions, ribs, and other tissues to allow access to deeper parts of the body.

Retrieval bag A sterile bag that is inserted into the body during minimally invasive surgery to aid the removal of tissues, such as the gallbladder. Use of a retrieval bag helps to avoid contamination of the wound with, for example, bile or infected tissues.

Scalpel A small knife with a sharp, disposable blade, used for cutting during surgery.

Spinal anesthesia A form of local anesthetic in which drugs are injected directly into the cerebrospinal fluid surrounding the spinal cord.

Spinal stenosis Narrowing of the spinal canal to compress the spinal cord or spinal nerves.

Staple A metal clip used to close a wound after surgery.

Stent An artificial tube inserted into a passage within the body to hold it open and reduce narrowing. Stents are most commonly inserted into a coronary artery.

Stoma An opening that connects part of a body cavity to the outside. A surgical procedure that produces a stoma is indicated with the suffix -ostomy, e.g. colostomy, ileostomy. The mouth is an example of a natural stoma.

Suction tube A drainage tube used to remove body fluids, such as amniotic fluid during cesarean section.

Suture A surgical stitch.

Swabs Sterile, gauze squares used to clean wounds, absorb blood, and help maintain a clear view of the operative field during surgery.

Thyroid gland An endocrine gland found at the base of the neck, in the front.

Thyroidectomy Removal of all or part of the thyroid gland.

Tissue A group of specialized cells with similar properties that come together to carry out a specific function. There are four main types of tissue in the body: muscle tissue, epithelial tissue, connective tissue, and nervous tissue.

Tonsillectomy Surgical removal of the tonsils.

Tonsillitis Inflammation of the tonsils.

Tonsils Lymph tissue found on either side of the throat, at the back.

Tourniquet A tight band applied to stop the flow of blood within a limb, e.g. during carpal tunnel surgery.

Umbilical cord The cord connecting a developing baby to the placenta, which is clamped and cut during cesarean section and normal delivery.

Vein A type of blood vessel that carries blood toward the heart. All veins, except for the pulmonary veins (and the umbilical vein during pregnancy), carry de-oxygenated blood.

Vermiform appendix A worm-like, blind-ending structure that branches off from the first part of the large bowel.

INDEX

Page numbers in **bold** denote a
main entry

Text by Dr Sarah Brewer
Edited by Philip de Ste. Croix
Designed by Paul Turner and Sue Pressley, Stonecastle Graphics Ltd
Index by Harry Sharp

Picture credits:
a = above, b = below, r = right, l = left

All pictures © Medicimage (www.medicimage.co.uk),
with the exception of the following:

© Science Photo Library: 105*(a)*; AJ Photo 103, 104*(l)*; Dr M.A. Ansary 104*(r)*;
Samuel Ashfield 51; John Bavosi 53; Biophoto Associates 54*(al)*; Colin Cuthbert
151*(b)*, 153*(a)*; Bsip Edwige 102; Michelle Del Guercio, Peter Arnold Inc.
120*(a)*; Dr Najeeb Layyous 136*(al)*; Dr P. Marazzi 118*(br)*, 119, 120*(b)*, 129*(al)*,
150, 151*(a)*, 153*(b)*; Arno Massee 121; Mr Gordon Muir / Consultant Urological
Surgeon / Renaissance Healthcare Ltd 144; Mr Gordon Muir / Tony McConnell
142, 143*(a)*, 143*(b)*; Louise Oligny 47*(a)*; Antonia Reeve 48*(a)*, 48*(b)*, 49;
Mark Thomas 57; Jim Varney 56*(a)*; Zephyr 126*(br)*, 127.

© Shutterstock.com: Simone van den Berg 38, 59; Brasiliao 1;
Monkey Business Images 123; Sherry Yates Sowell 155.

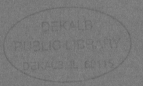